The Right Thing

· ·

Emily Friedman

· ·

Foreword by Kathryn E. Johnson

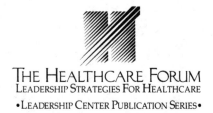

THE HEALTHCARE FORUM
LEADERSHIP STRATEGIES FOR HEALTHCARE
•LEADERSHIP CENTER PUBLICATION SERIES•

The Right Thing

Ten Years of Ethics Columns
from the *Healthcare
Forum Journal*

Jossey-Bass Publishers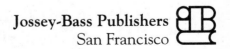
San Francisco

Substantial discounts on bulk quantities of Jossey-Bass books are available to corporations, professional associations, and other organizations. For details and discount information, contact the special sales department at Jossey-Bass Inc., Publishers (415) 433-1740; Fax (800) 605-2665.

For sales outside the United States, please contact your local Simon & Schuster International Office.

 Manufactured in the United States of America on Lyons Falls Pathfinder Tradebook. This paper is acid-free and 100 percent totally chlorine-free.

Library of Congress Cataloging-in-Publication Data

Friedman, Emily.
   The right thing : ten years of ethics columns from the Healthcare forum journal / Emily Friedman.
     p. cm.
   Includes bibliographical references and index.
   ISBN 0-7879-0225-X
   1. Medical ethics. I. Healthcare forum journal. II. Title.
R724.F75   1996
174'.2—dc20
                                96–3295

PB Printing   10 9 8 7 6 5 4 3 2 1   FIRST EDITION

Contents

· ·

For
Em Jay, John G., and Ginger
Judy, Libby, Don, and Herk
Herb and Betty
Dorothy, Wes, and Rex

My early friends, "family," and mentors,
who taught me more about ethical and compassionate behavior
than any university could

Foreword

Kathryn E. Johnson

As a writer, lecturer, and health policy and ethics analyst, Emily Friedman has the unique talent of translating healthcare statistics and ethics into a language we can easily relate to and apply to our personal and professional lives.

As a contributing editor to the *Healthcare Forum Journal* and author of the *Journal*'s feature column "Making Choices," Emily consistently delivers a timely, thought-provoking editorial on a broad spectrum of healthcare issues. She brings the perspectives of a diverse group to the forefront—be it patient, practitioner, community, or government—and she leaves us with a better understanding and appreciation for all concerned from all the angles.

It is no small coincidence that her feature is placed at the beginning of each issue of the *Healthcare Forum Journal*. Setting the stage for each edition's theme, Emily continually challenges us to:

- Open our minds and hearts to the stories that follow.

- Share and learn from our experiences.

- Gain insight into the ever-evolving world of healthcare.

- Remember that behind the statistics are real people requiring compassion (lest we forget that when we talk about "them," we are also talking about "us").

Through her "Making Choices" column over the past decade, Emily has helped readers explore trends and changes in healthcare delivery, the wisdom of our decisions, and the ethical issues implicit in our complex industry. And here we bring you a collection of many of those thought-provoking, challenging columns. We'll travel into the future of community-based health planning, envision the impact of global technology, and examine the removal of barriers to healthcare as we venture into the twenty-first century.

Acknowledgments

In early 1986, I was only a few months past quitting my job and entering the sometimes wonderful world of free-lance writing. I had published three pieces in *Healthcare Forum* (later *Healthcare Forum Journal*): a rewrite of a speech I had given in 1983, an article on women in healthcare administration, and a piece on healthcare consumerism. The journal's editor, Susan Anthony, invited me to lunch at a restaurant in the Emporium Capwell department store in San Francisco (the things one remembers!). During that lunch, she asked if I would be interested in writing a column for the journal. I suggested doing something on health services research; she said she would prefer that I write one on ethics. She thought it would reach more readers. She was, I suspect, right, as Susan is about many things. So now it can be told: "Making Choices," for better or worse, is all Sue Anthony's fault.

A few other people can share the blame, among them Kathryn Johnson, long-time leader of the Forum, who has welcomed my sometimes-inflammatory writing ever since we met in Yosemite in 1983; and two editors who continued to support the column during the years between Sue's departure and return, Jeff Brown and Ellen Jo Bayliss. Three other true editorial professionals—Judith Jenna, Lance Levy, and Susan Sasenick—have for years found and fixed my boo-boos, edited my prose, and kept the process on track, despite my penchant for slightly missing deadlines. I wish that non-publishing people knew how critical editors are to the writer and the quality of his or her work!

In terms of this book, I owe a great debt of gratitude, again, to Sue Anthony, as well as to Gayle Samuelson of the Healthcare Forum, who has done most of the frustrating logistical and diplomatic work on the project, and to Becky McGovern and Michele Hubinger of Jossey-Bass.

Finally, I would like to thank those people who got me into the ethics biz to begin with, and who continue to serve as mentors and guides: George Annas, Audrey Kaufman, Rudolf Klein, Alan Sager, Dorothy Saxner, Judith Swazey, and the many others who plough through the swamps in search of the right thing. Maybe someday we'll find it.

E.F.

Introduction

I began writing the "Making Choices" column in early 1986. At that time, Ronald Reagan was President of the United States and Republicans controlled the Senate (they would lose that control in the November 1986 election); Democrats controlled the House of Representatives. Congress that year would allow the health planning law to expire (to the relief of almost everyone except the planning agencies); there were 29,003 documented cases of AIDS in this country; Medicare said it would begin to cover heart transplants at certain designated centers; Surgeon General C. Everett Koop, M.D., was making waves.

In biomedical ethics, among the hot issues were abortion rights; AIDS; organ transplantation; the "Baby Doe" rule (federal regulations requiring that care be provided to even profoundly compromised newborns, regardless of potential quantity or quality of life); ethics committees; using anencephalic newborns (infants born with no brain) as organ donors; and various right-to-die issues.

Any of that sound familiar?

Nearly ten years later, it is interesting that certain issues remain with us in their full heat, whereas others seem to have been settled or at least to have calmed down. Among the still white-hot concerns are abortion, AIDS, and some aspects of organ transplantation. We do not hear so much about ethics committees, which are old (if still good) news, or about Baby Doe rules. The reason for lack of controversy over the former is that ethics committees have become part of the furniture, something that we expect to have around; the reason for lack of controversy over the latter is that the "Baby Doe" regulations have long since been overturned by the courts—and they were more an ideological political issue than a healthcare issue in the first place.

The Democrats came back to control both houses of Congress (at least until 1994), and a Democrat was elected president in 1992. Because Democrats tend to support abortion rights, the federal government stopped trying to limit access to abortion the way it had under Republican administrations. Furthermore, in several measured decisions, the Supreme Court upheld the rights of states to circumscribe access to abortion in various ways—but not to outlaw the procedure.

A look back at the ethics literature of 1986 is also instructive in terms of what it does not include. There is no mention of physician-assisted suicide or xenografts (transplantation of organs from animals to human beings); nor is there mention of the 35 million or so people who were uninsured that year, or of the ethical implications of capitation and managed care.

There was some discussion of for-profit enterprise in healthcare, but no one had heard of Columbia/HCA (which did not then exist, although HCA did as a separate firm) or many of the proprietary health maintenance organizations that have since risen to prominence.

This look back at the past ten years provides us with at least three lessons that I find compelling. The first is that although sincere and sometimes heroic effort on the part of providers, ethicists, policymakers, and just plain folks can bring about consensus on some issues—the case of Karen Quinlan and its enormous impact on the ability of people to die as they choose comes to mind—other issues are so intractable that there is really very little hope that we will come to terms on them. The paradigm issue is, of course, abortion; although most Americans are somewhere in the middle, the most influential and vocal positions are held by those who are either totally against it or totally for it, and they are unlikely to move toward middle ground. Indeed, the fact that murders have been committed in the name of the anti-abortion cause would lead one to believe that the two sides are moving farther apart.

Other issues are likely to be just as stubborn: Seeking donor organs from living siblings or parents; xenografts; euthanasia. It is not just that the issues are difficult; it is that they are enmeshed in multiple layers of deeply held beliefs, political ideologies, fears, hopes, and exploitation, and it is virtually impossible to strip all that away and get down to the basic ideas that should be at the heart of the debate.

The second lesson is that ethics is perceived by the person on the street as an arcane discipline whose practitioners dwell in ivory towers and debate the number of organ transplants you can do on the head of a pin. Ethics is seen as something pure and above the political fray. But the fact is that many critical ethics issues have been thoroughly politicized, never so much as in the past 20 years and especially the last 10. Abortion issues became entangled with hydration, nutrition, and patients' unwritten wishes in the *Cruzan* case; questions of coercion and informed consent became entangled with questions of organ transplantation; questions of patients' right to die "with dignity" became entangled with questions of euthanasia; questions of advance directives became entangled with questions of cost containment.

What started out as ethics issues became quandaries for providers and moved from there into courts, legislatures, and Congress. The next thing we knew, federal law required providers to ask patients if they would like to donate their organs in case they did not survive their healthcare experience; federal law also mandated that providers offer patients information about living wills and other advanced directives. Even the Clinton health care reform task force of 1993 had an ethics advisory group, although its recommendations seem to have been studiously ignored, and the supposed "ethics principles" of the Clinton plan had little to do with morality or justice.

This politicization of basic human questions of life and death, this turning of delicate and complex issues into ham-handed legislation, this transformation of profound beliefs into ideological combat, gives me the creeps. But that's how things are just now.

The third lesson is much more cheering, at least to me: the expansion, in the past 10 years, of ethics past the cult of the individual. If the paradigms of 1986 were narrow issues of individual rights, today at least some of the paradigms have to do with lack of access to care, rationing, managed care, profiteering, and the like. This is long overdue. When Judith Swazey and Renee Fox first stated in 1984 that there was a difference between "medical morality" (which they defined as providers behaving in an acceptable way toward patients) and bioethics (which they defined as the promulgation of moral principles that could and should apply to all of healthcare and to society itself), not too many ethicists paid much attention. Indeed, some members of the bioethics community thought that those who were interested in social ethics, as opposed to individual ethics, were way out of line.

However, somewhere along the way, the bioethics community learned that the individual ethics bone is connected to the societal ethics bone; that the poet John Donne was right when he said no man is an island. Today, the ethics net is cast wide enough to recognize 43 million uninsured Americans, inappropriate constraint on access practiced by some HMOs, and wild maldistribution of healthcare resources as true ethics problems.

There are other areas in which those who pursue ethics may take satisfaction. Processes are now in place in most healthcare organizations—encouraged by law, regulation, accreditation requirements and even a bit of a young tradition—that provide forums (usually ethics committees) where providers, patients, families, and sometimes even representatives of the community can hash out difficult questions of all kinds, and, one hopes, come to consensus.

There is now much more discussion among front-line providers—physicians, nurses, and others who do the work of patient care—about issues that trouble them. No longer is unilateral, undiscussed, often secret decision making the order of the day; health care folk feel more comfortable asking peers for advice and consultation.

There is much more collaboration between patient and physician, patient and nurse, and physician and nurse. The paternalistic model of "Me Doctor–You Patient" has largely disappeared, although it hangs on, often in the most inopportune circumstances. Patients can express their wishes, can challenge physicians, can ask for clinical data, can choose from more options. Although this form of decision making is not always easy for physicians and nurses who believe they know the best thing to do, it allows patients to be something more than helpless pawns in a system they do not understand, and few can argue with that.

But things are not entirely rosy in Ethics Land. It is true that we have been able to move from the strictly individual situation to include the social situation as well. It is true that we have resolved many aspects of several troubling issues, most notably those involving patients' rights and patients' ability to set the terms of their own deaths. But there is much more work to do.

We must find a way to disentangle ethics issues from political agendas, whether they be on the Right or on the Left, so that the fragile interconnections that represent the healthcare experience are not fractured by a hail of bullets from outsiders who really have no interest in the specific situation—only in the political hay to be made.

We must find a way to develop acceptable rules of the road for the new challenges that lie down the thoroughfare that opens up to healthcare at the end of the 21st century: Technologies that can succeed, but that can also fail, with results that are horrific and costly beyond imagination; the information revolution, which promises a truly integrated, interactive medical record and healthcare history that can greatly improve healthcare quality, but that also offers the threat that a sixth-grade student who is a competent computer hacker can learn even the most intimate details of a patient's life; and the ever-present issue of how to allocate health-care resources in the most fair fashion—no small job in a nation where healthcare entrepreneurs make hundreds of millions of dollars in one year, and half our children go about unimmunized.

Finally, bioethics itself faces some daunting challenges. Flush with early success in areas such as living wills and patients' right to refuse treatment, healthcare ethics has exploded into an industry. Everywhere there are ethics centers, ethics conferences, ethics newsletters, ethics books (including this one), ethics consulting services. I have no doubt that ethicists and ethics firms will soon join providers in slugging it out for managed care contracts. Perhaps the result of those contracts will be a new concept: managed ethics.

Healthcare ethics and the people who toil in its vineyards have at least three special rows to hoe:

First, bioethics remains too academic and distant from the trenches of healthcare. Most ethicists have never cared for a patient or worked in a hospital or clinic or HMO. Although ethics does require the luxury of distance, I have become tired of ethics analysts who, working only in the realm of the theoretical, either promulgate pretty plans that cannot possibly work in the real healthcare world, or else reject more pragmatic approaches because somewhere, at some time, some one case might come up to which the approach might not apply.

Second, the bioethics community is still not influential enough. Yes, legislation and regulation and television shows address ethics concerns, but all too often that is the result of individual patients and their families bringing their traumas to television. Ethics journals and newsletters and conferences play a crucial role in identifying and debating issues, but it is not their scholarly ruminations that make the news and influence policymakers; it is Jack Kevorkian and Mickey Mantle. Bioethicists should spend a little less time on the seductive but nonetheless self-limiting practice of talking to themselves and each other, and a bit more time on trying to get their message out to everybody else.

Third and finally, everyone in healthcare needs to learn that ethics is not an offshoot of alchemy or witchcraft; it is simply learning to do one's job, and to provide service to others, in a manner that is comfortable, given what one thinks are the rights and wrongs of this world. Ethics principles are not frills, or petticoats, or appendixes on the body of healthcare; they are the ultimate determinant of whether what we do, and how we do it, will be acceptable in the eyes of our people. For the practice of ethics, in the end, is rooted in a recognition of the most basic principle of all: Actions have consequences.

If John Donne was right—and he was—then he was the first bioethicist. For it was he who wrote:

> Any man's death diminishes me, because I am
> involved in mankind; and therefore never send
> to know for whom the bell tolls; it tolls for
> thee.

February 1996   Emily Friedman
                                                         Chicago, Illinois

Organ Transplants

A Lesson from Canada

July 1986

*This was my first "Making Choices" column.
Although it is quite outdated—the Canadian healthcare system, like our own, has changed a very great
deal—we are including it here for, shall we say, "historical interest." Besides, the principles promulgated
by the task force remain highly relevant, especially
in this country, which continues to have far too
many transplant programs and an escalating number
of controversies concerning organ transplantation.*

As healthcare becomes more sophisticated, pathways that were once clearly demarcated grow treacherous. One ethical minefield is care that is expensive, difficult, often underfunded, and involves use of scarce resources. Many of these forms of care are effective—but only under certain circumstances. This puts provider, payer, and regulator alike to the test in a delicately balanced decision-making process.

Organ transplants are a highly visible example. Among the issues they raise are: Who should receive them? Who should provide them? Who should pay for them? How can organs be ethically obtained, distributed, and used? What are the respective roles of government and the private sector? Who should make the rules?

In the United States, several organizations, particularly the Department of Health and Human Services Task Force on Organ Transplantation, have been wrestling with these issues. In Canada, however, a transplant policy developed by the Working Group on Vital Organ Transplant Centres is being implemented. It could provide some guidance for American policy.

These are the major conclusions of the Canadian task force:

1. Organ transplantation is "effective and acceptable" when compared with other, comparable therapies.

2. "A sufficient supply of organs is potentially available to meet demand in 1990."

3. "Organ transplantation should be viewed, not as an isolated program, but in the broader context of end-stage organ failure programs." (Transplantation is often more cost-effective than other forms of therapy, even though the one-time expenditure may be significant. However, the report recommends that transplant programs be funded through trade-offs of existing funds, rather than through the infusion of large amounts of new money.)

4. Transplant programs should be provincial or regional, with mobile transplant teams, rather than being "owned" by individual hospitals.

5. Programs should be based only in teaching centers where proper personnel and technical expertise are already available. (The report further recommends minimum volumes of procedures per center, and opposes development of new programs until all existing programs have reached minimum volume levels.)

6. Provincial health authorities should decide on issues such as the cost of transportation of donor organs and/or recipients to the transplant center, coverage of the costs of acquisition of organs, definitions of brain death, and protection of the rights of donors.

7. Currently available information on transplants is not sufficient to allow proper monitoring and evaluation over the
   long term, and better information gathering is necessary.

None of these proposals is revolutionary; in fact, many of
them are similar to the recommendations made by the organ
transplant task force in Massachusetts in 1984. The difference is
that the Massachusetts report ran into political trouble, and many
of its recommendations were ignored. The Canadian report is
being implemented.

Two policy areas that the Canadian document addresses are particularly difficult for American policymakers. One is the cost versus access equation—the issue of rationing and resource allocation.
The report notes that "in almost all areas of consideration, the conclusions and recommendations were reached by compromising
between two factors—quality of care and costs of care." The working group adds, "If the number of transplants is to be increased in
the future, one must consider the extent to which government goals
of cost containment and quality of care will be challenged or dollars will be diverted from other forms of health programming. [This]
is one of the most difficult ethical problems posed by funding of a
service such as organ transplantation."

The report concludes that despite the effectiveness of transplants, the programs "will have to demonstrate to the public" that
their benefits justify the expenditures involved.

The working group also observes that in Canada, allocation of
transplants and of organs is based on a combination of ethical criteria, including "medical success, medical neediness, and queuing."
The working group rejects age (except where prognosis is poor) and
income status as criteria.

Although this approach can be debated, it is certainly more
equitable and responsible than the hit-or-miss approach in the
United States—where often no criteria other than market factors
and press interest are used.

The other issue is standards for transplant programs. The Canadian panel members were willing to bite the bullet and say that the number of transplant centers should be restricted, that criteria for designating centers should be tough, and that minimal volume levels are important for ensuring high-quality programs. The report defines "desirable" annual transplant volume per center as 50 for kidneys, 20 for livers, 30 for hearts, and 36 for bone marrow. The panel found insufficient evidence for pancreas and heart/lung transplants, which they consider experimental.

American planners have not been so disposed. For example, although the National Heart Transplantation Study, conducted by the Battelle Human Affairs Research Centers for HCFA, provided persuasive evidence that 20 heart transplants per year per center are optimal to ensure quality, transplant centers in the United States continue to proliferate beyond estimated statistical need.

Developing this report was undoubtedly a difficult task for the clinicians and regulators involved. They stress their concerns about ethics, access, fairness, and policy flexibility throughout the report. But at least they were willing to take the stand that quality and the protection of the patient, rather than institutional or clinical ego, should determine the future of transplantation. Let us hope that American policy planners show equal courage.

. . . .

Whose Responsibility Is It, Anyway?

September 1986

There is a burgeoning interest these days in healthcare ethicists: people skilled in the theory and practice of ethics, who provide advice, counsel, and information to patients, families, and hospital staff. The demand is so great that some organizations keep rosters of ethicists in order to answer inquiries from prospective employers.

I think that hospital ethicists are needed—just as they are needed in healthcare systems, health maintenance organizations, nursing homes (especially), and other settings. With the difficult problems facing providers, it is invaluable to have the counsel of someone who knows how people have dealt with similar dilemmas in the past, what the current experience is, how value systems can shape and be shaped by their environments as well as the best means of pursuing "the right thing." When it comes to termination of treatment, care for the medically indigent, appropriate care for the dying, and sorting out who is right when families, patients, and physicians disagree, we need all the help we can get.

There are problems, however. One is conflicts over turf. Educated in the ethics of their professions and confronted by ethical dilemmas on a daily basis, clinical and pastoral care professionals often do not like the idea of someone else being selected as the source of all ethical knowledge.

It's like the "designated hitter" in baseball who waltzes in to hit but does not have to play in the field, inning after inning. But once it is clear that the ethicist is there to help others sort out their own decisions and values, rather than to tell them what to do, the conflict usually subsides.

Does Having an Ethicist Mean You're Ethical?

The other problem is that too many people at the hospital see that an ethicist has been hired and say, "Well, that's taken care of." If an institution has an ethicist it must be ethical, so we can forget about that and go back to the wars. This attitude can be reinforced by the fact that many hospital employees do not ever come into contact with the ethicist or the institutional ethics program.

Hiring an ethicist should be viewed not as an end in itself but rather as the beginning of a process. This process should culminate in an active, ongoing, system-wide ethics program—and in a commitment from all those involved with the hospital to ensure the institution conducts itself in an ethical manner.

"Don't be silly," you say. "Of course we're ethical. We provide healthcare!" But is that always the case? Ethicist Carl Middleton, of the Sisters of Charity of the Incarnate Word in Houston, makes the point that although individual patient care issues are critical, it is the ongoing processes and policies of an institution that test its ethics. Hospital managers, he says, can profess the highest of ethics—and then "budget like barbarians."

Sister Melanie Di Pietro, a Pittsburgh attorney, echoes Middleton's view. At a Catholic Health Corporation meeting last Spring, she observed that a hospital's policies and procedures were the truest indicators of allegiance to its ethical mission. She asked, for example, "to whom does the hospital provide free parking—patients, housekeepers, or physicians?"

I often ask hospital managers, when they lament the indigent care problem, what provisions they have made for health insurance coverage for the employees they have laid off.

The Growing Isolation

Even if a provider is ethically committed, it's difficult to spread the word to all employees. There are so many of them, a large number of whom are not involved in direct patient care; many also work the "off" shifts. Furthermore, they do not have as much contact with each other as did their predecessors. Mitch Rabkin, MD, president of Beth Israel Hospital in Boston, points out that the computer has severed many of the channels through which hospital employees used to get to know each other.

When I worked at the Kaiser Foundation Hospital in Oakland, California, I delivered lab report slips throughout the hospital and was in frequent contact with patients, physicians, nurses, ward clerks, and others. Rabkin observes, "Today, we glance at a computer screen for test results; the folks in the lab are faceless and unknown. That does not help produce a sense of community."

Also, staffing patterns are leaner now, which cuts down on the amount of time even direct care givers can spend on ethical niceties. Nurses, in particular, complain about not having the time to chat with patients about hobbies or look at pictures of the grandchildren. The length of stay is too short, and the workload is too heavy. Who has time for ethics or mission?

Things have changed for trustees as well. Traditionally, women trustees, especially, were often in touch with patients as volunteers and auxiliaries. Now trustees complain that they have been removed from any patient contact. A prominent trustee said recently, "I never get to visit patients anymore, and patients are what a hospital is supposed to be about. *They* are why I'm a trustee."

Hiring an ethicist won't diminish this growing sense of isolation. The leadership has to come from higher up: from the board and from the medical staff. After all, trustees hold ultimate responsibility for the institution: It is they who must set policy. As Paul Hofmann, executive director of Emory University Hospital in

Atlanta and chairman of the AHA Special Committee on Bio-medical Ethics, has said, "The board is the institutional conscience of the hospital."

Physicians are the guardians of the quality of care in the insti-tution, although I believe that nursing professionals share that charge. Ethical commitment and behavior are part of the provision of high-quality care. And physicians have been trained in ethics, and have taken an oath to honor that training. We can all point to doctors who have fallen down on the job, but overall I think physi-cians can exercise powerful ethical leadership.

Whether or not a healthcare provider hires an ethicist, it needs to make an *institutional* commitment to ethics. This means (1) *spe-cific* board and medical staff consideration of ethics problems and priorities, (2) policy development, and (3) participatory discussion of the ethical responsibilities of hospital managers and other employ-ees in light of that policy. How an ethics program can be imple-mented at the individual employee level must be determined as well.

No matter what is decided in the room of the terminally ill patient, and no matter what the official indigent care policy is, if its employees think ethics are someone else's department, then the hospital has not done its job.

. . . .

Decisions and Default

November 1986

I s being involved in the provision of healthcare an ethical good, in and of itself? If you are a physician, nurse, hospital manager, or trustee, are you safe in assuming that because you do what you do, you are conducting yourself in an ethical manner? It's surprising how many healthcare professionals will answer "yes."

I don't think they're right. Why? Because many morally and ethically wrong things can and do occur in healthcare, *if someone doesn't prevent them from happening.* There are times when not taking action may be the right thing to do. But *not doing something* can, in fact, constitute a grievous moral wrong.

In the policy arena, for example, a non-action that resulted in harm was what several state Medicaid programs did not do during the ruinous inflation of the Seventies. They simply did not adjust income levels for welfare eligibility to reflect inflation. Although the working poor were still losing ground in terms of real income, they found their wages rising. Many of these people became ineligible for welfare and Medicaid. Voila! Poor people who used to be "deserving" were suddenly disenfranchised, and Medicaid rolls were reduced—without the policymakers having to lift a finger.

Looking the Other Way

In the hospital, the same sort of thing can take place. Let's say the medical staff uses the first-come, first-served approach to admitting patients to a crowded coronary care unit. The administration says that's fine. But the administration doesn't ever check to make sure that this system is working. And, as Tristram Engelhardt, MD, pointed out in the March 7, 1986 issue of the *Journal of the American Medical Association*, the first-come, first-served approach, when it isn't monitored, has its drawbacks.

He cites the case of Susan Von Stetina, an auto accident victim who was admitted to an overflowing intensive care unit and suffered severe permanent brain damage because there was insufficient ICU staff to give her proper attention. The hospital lost the resulting lawsuit, in part because it was shown that one of the other ICU patients was effectively brain dead and two others were discharged from the hospital the next morning. Yet nobody did anything to transfer these patients—who were obviously in less need of ICU care than Von Stetina—to another unit in the hospital. Here, inaction was found to be a legal as well as a moral wrong.

Then there's the continuing reluctance of physicians, nurses, and other clinical professionals to "blow the whistle" on fellow practitioners who are incompetent, impaired, or unprofessional. Even the threat of malpractice litigation is not enough to spur a doctor or nurse to prevent another doctor or nurse from harming patients. We read of a surgeon who raped anesthetized patients in the surgical suite; yet no one seems to have noticed. How could you *not* notice? We read of physicians performing surgery while obviously drunk—while everyone looks the other way.

News reports cite "standing orders" in some hospitals to send unstabilized, critically ill, medically indigent patients to some other hospital—in a taxicab! A hospital association professional once advised emergency department managers to set up a separate waiting room for the poor—one with no chairs in it. None of this is ethically or even professionally defensible; yet, because these are not actions, but non-actions, people feel more comfortable with them.

Avoiding Scary Decisions

We are more inclined to accept inaction, I think, because Americans tend to default in the face of painful decisions. For example, I believe we have surrendered much of our privacy and sense of self-protection (and often common sense) to physicians because we want them to make scary decisions for us.

In the policy arena, the United States has long exercised health policy by default, with less global issues (usually variants on the themes of cost, quality, and access) taking turns serving as the basis of policy decisions. In both micro and macro areas of healthcare, our most common response appears to be avoidance. Thus, for the individual or institutional caregiver, why not do the same when it comes to the ethics of what one does?

Ethicist Albert Jonsen, Ph.D., points out that we condemn *commission* far more than we do *omission*. We are harsher on the wrong committed *intentionally* than on the wrong committed *unintentionally*. We are less forgiving when the *ordinary*, the *expected*, act is not committed than we are if the *extraordinary* is not done. And, as anyone involved in termination of treatment will attest, we find *stopping* care worse than *not starting* it.

In all these instances, the idea seems to be that you're going to get clobbered more for doing something consciously than for allowing something to happen. Therefore, most people choose the path of default. It is the ultimate expression of the oft-repeated hope that "if we ignore it, maybe it will go away."

The problem, of course, is that avoiding ethical analysis of one's actions and their consequences doesn't mean that bad things won't happen. Just because we refuse to take an action or to consider its consequences does not mean that the action will not be taken or the consequences will not occur. Furthermore, in this litigious country, people are held legally responsible for what they did not do, or for what they allowed to happen, as much as they are held responsible for actions they knowingly undertook—as the *Von Stetina* case showed.

The legal definition of sanity in the United States is being able to recognize and understand the consequences of one's own actions. I think that definition applies, not only to one's mental health, but to one's ethical health.

There is no such thing as automatic ethics. And I do not believe that anyone can work in healthcare, *in any capacity*, and make morally defensible decisions by default. Decisions must be conscious and their results recognized. If you initiate a heart transplant program when you know that you will likely only perform three or four transplants a year, you should fully understand the consequences—social, quality, clinical, financial, and other—of that action. If you ignore the problem of an incompetent physician on the staff, you should realize the probable results of that choice.

Conscious Ethical Choices

How does one combat default and avoidance? First, establish a baseline of accountability. Ask yourself, **Whom do I serve?** Everyone has more than one answer—my patients, my hospital, the public, my community, my stockholders, my employees. List the answers in order of priority, so you are clear about where your first responsibilities lie.

The second question is either **Why am I afraid to make a conscious decision on this issue?** or **Why am I unwilling to think about the consequences of this decision?** It may be that you are avoiding one or the other because of an ethical conflict you would rather not confront (it will help the bottom line but some patients will suffer).

Third, **What will be the consequences of my decision?** Ask this about each of the options involved in a complex choice.

Fourth, and perhaps most important, ask the question we don't ask often enough: **What will be the consequences of my not making a decision?** Through this exercise, we come to understand that default is a blind—that, in fact, not to decide is to decide. But through this exercise we also establish an ethical *process* that, if properly and regularly pursued when difficult issues surface, will more than likely produce an ethical *outcome*.

Of Providers and Plagues

January 1987

This was the first of three columns I have written about AIDS, the plague of our time. (The other two, also in this volume, were "AIDS and Insurers: Keeping the Covenant?" and "The Toad at the Edge of the World.") At the time of its writing—the end of 1986—I was distressed because 15,000 Americans had died of the disease. Nearly ten years later, at the end of 1995, more than 300,000 were dead in this country; more than 1 million had been infected. Back when I wrote this, the largest patient populations were gay men, intravenous drug users, and, it was thought, Caribbean immigrants (which turned out not to be true, but we Americans really seem to have it in for Haitians). Now the fastest-growing population is heterosexual young people. But because gay men and minorities are still disproportionately represented, the disease is often considered to be someone else's problem. Indeed, Senator Jesse Helms (R-North Carolina) recently tried to stop funding under the Ryan White AIDS law, which pays for treatment of patients, because he considers persons with AIDS to deserve their fate. Insurers in most states can still discriminate against those with HIV, Medicaid continues to be the largest third-party payer of AIDS costs, and the flower of our youth continue to die.

A s I write this, at least 15,000 persons in this country have died from AIDS. Another 25,000 are afflicted. Estimates are that between 1 and 1.5 million Americans are at risk of going down the same one-way street; at least 250,000 of them may die.

Over a glass of wine, a friend of mine—a male homosexual in San Francisco—takes issue with me when I say that homosexuals tend to get the cancer while intravenous drug users get the pneumonia. "I don't think so," he says calmly, dispassionately. "Most of my friends who have died had the pneumonia." *Most of his friends who have died.* This man is not yet 30. He should not have reason to talk about the wholesale loss of friends to natural causes.

But is acquired immune deficiency syndrome a "natural cause"? Some say it is not, that it is the wrath of God, visited upon those who have sinned. After all, they say, look at who gets it: male homosexuals with multiple sexual partners, prostitutes, intravenous drug users, some low-income black immigrants. There are others, of course: people (mostly hemophiliacs) who are infected through blood transfusion, and sexual partners of infected individuals of either sex.

If it's a punishment for unpopular lifestyles, I don't understand why junkies get it and "crack" users don't; nor can I come up with a good reason why being a hemophiliac or being poor and black is a sin. Furthermore, I have yet to meet a virus that thinks, let alone makes decisions about the relative social worth of the owner of the cells it attacks. No, I think AIDS is something far more mindless.

Our reaction to it is sometimes equally mindless. In the individual patient, the disease attacks the immune system. In society, what the disease appears to be attacking is our common sense and our humanity. And many of these battles are being played out in the American healthcare system.

The plague mentality is nothing new. Bubonic plague killed about 75 million Europeans between 1347 and 1351. Epidemiology was not the strong point of those cultures, so they sought other reasons for the catastrophe. As has often been the case, many people decided the Jews were responsible (gypsies are also a popular target in such situations) and quite a few Jews were burned alive.

In 1831, a cholera epidemic led Hungarian peasants to revolt, claiming that the aristocracy was trying to kill them so they wouldn't revolt. (Needless to say, if that was the intent, the strategy didn't work very well.)

Assailed from Both Sides

During the dreadful influenza epidemic in the United States in 1918–1919, uniformed public health nurses in Philadelphia were subject to two distinct threats. On the one hand, the sick besieged them on the street, begging for help. On the other hand, healthy people shunned them, fearing that the nurses carried the disease. In times of plague, healthcare providers are assailed from both sides.

It is no different today. On the one hand, AIDS victims can count on hospitals and physicians to care for them, even if those providers tend to be in the public sector (at least when it comes to undocumented Haitian immigrants, IV drug users, and others unlikely to have heath insurance). And some AIDS sufferers have been allowed to continue their duties as hospital employees.

On the other hand, it was a sad day when the first employer charged by the federal government with violating the rights of an AIDS-afflicted employee was a hospital. And we are all familiar with instances in which hospital employees refused to touch or provide care to victims of AIDS.

One enterprising Californian seeking high political office proposed that hospital employees be allowed to wear any kind of protective clothing they chose when treating AIDS patients. (One wonders how a dying, terrified patient would react when approached by a nurse in a beekeeper's suit.)

Another California proposal would have required all donated blood to be labeled as to the gender of the donor; the sponsor reasoned that because women don't get AIDS (which is hardly the case), the wise transfusion recipient would demand only blood donated by women.

This sort of stupidity aside, there are many serious questions. How can healthcare providers confront the ethical aspects of this tragedy? It's a little tricky when you're wrestling with protecting the blood supply, ensuring the rights of patients and employees, trying to protect the confidentiality of test results, grappling with insufficient funding for the care of AIDS patients, and trying to provide compassionate and meaningful care for those patients.

Even the attorney who sued the city of New York over the presence of children with AIDS in the classroom had second thoughts. "You know," he said later, "40 percent of the time, I think the children should be allowed in school. Another 40 percent of the time, I think they should be kept at home. And 20 percent of the time, I don't know what I think."

Suggestions for Coping

When conflicting rights and values all have merit, there are no sure answers. However, here are a few guidelines to use in dealing with practical AIDS ethics:

Try to fight hysteria and misinformation. No care giver, institutional or individual, should allow an environment of bigotry and terror to develop in the healthcare setting. We know enough about this disease to keep employees and patients properly informed about risk.

You will not contract AIDS from a toilet seat. All gays, Haitians, junkies, and hookers are not AIDS victims. It is not dangerous to work in the same place with an AIDS sufferer, nor, with reasonable precautions, is it dangerous to care for them. Most of us have probably unknowingly worked alongside someone who has the virus, and most hospital employees have probably cared for such a person.

Encourage respect for and confidentiality of AIDS data. Leaked test results have serious consequences: loss of employment, loss of health insurance benefits, loss of friends or even family.

Healthcare providers are supposed to honor the privacy of their patients *above all*. I don't recall any paragraphs in the Hippocratic oath or other professional codes of ethics that have an asterisk that indicates "except in the case of AIDS."

Have some sensitivity and savvy when conducting educational efforts. We have approached health education not so much on the basis of helping potential victims as with the attitude that we don't want them to get their cooties on us. For example, the United States has been less than sympathetic with heroin addicts; yet we now tell them not to share needles because we're concerned that we might catch AIDS from them. I'm afraid we have given them little reason to want to protect us.

We tell IV drug users that they may harm their health if they share needles. Well, generally speaking, I don't think good health habits are a high priority for people who are injecting known toxins into their veins with dirty needles. If we can't develop an ethos of caring about high-risk populations *that involves more than our own self-interest*, I'm not sure how much good we will do.

Remember the fine line between "them" and "us." There is such a thing as "communitarian" ethics, which is the art of understanding that we are all in this together. One of the tragedies of AIDS is that, by and large, it affects disadvantaged populations who lie outside the mainstream of American society. It is this aspect of the disease that has allowed medieval attitudes to surface in a supposedly sophisticated age.

But AIDS is only one of many kinds of horrifying bad luck that can strike us. David Winston, one of the most powerful people in American healthcare, was killed in 1986 because he got into a quarrel with a truck driver on a public street. A woman was killed recently when she stepped out of a car at the side of a road just as a tire flew off a passing truck and struck her. People are victimized in lunatic, arbitrary ways. Today, for the tragic thousands, it is AIDS. Tomorrow, it could be something else, and it could be you or me. We must avoid breaking ourselves down into "them" and "us."

Kenneth Meeks, a gay activist and AIDS victim who died in 1986, was interviewed by Ted Koppel on "Nightline" as he lay dying in a hospital. The show had followed him for nearly a year, and it was an emotional moment for people on both sides of the camera. Koppel asked Meeks what he wanted to say for his last statement, which would be seen by millions of Americans.

"There are 240 million people calling themselves Americans, and there are 6 billion who call themselves human beings," Meeks replied. "I have an obligation to them—and they have an obligation to me." Let us fulfill that obligation by halting ignorance, cruelty, and bigotry at the healthcare provider's door.

Blaming the Victim

The Care Giver's Conflict

March 1987

It's a problem that arises for all people in healthcare, although it is more acute for physicians, nurses, and others who are in direct contact with patients: Some patients appear to be responsible for their own conditions. And when resources are scarce and other patients are the innocent victims of their ailments, it can be difficult to have much sympathy for patients who brought their troubles on through their own irresponsibility.

Among the patients who are most often the cause of such thoughts are those with substance abuse problems, traumatic injuries such as gunshot wounds sustained as a result of criminal activity, morbid obesity, problems brought on by cigarette smoking, and problems caused by knowing noncompliance with treatment regimens (such as diabetics who consume large amounts of alcohol).

At the same time, there are young children victimized by physical or emotional abuse, people who have been injured by drunken drivers, and elderly people who have been attacked on the street. There may be patients who have followed superb health practices all their lives only to be felled by multiple sclerosis or cancer. It's hard not to wonder why people who appear unworthy deserve equal—or even greater—amounts of healthcare than the innocent.

The conflict is between the care giver's commitment to providing care to all who come to her or him and the care giver's equally strong commitment to justice and the preservation of life.

How can anyone squander precious resources by abusing himself and then demanding that the healthcare system repair the damage? When life is so precious, how can anyone essentially commit suicide by smoking cigarettes or abusing alcohol?

Who "Deserves" Care?

There are several ways of confronting this conflict. One approach is to differentiate among patients in terms of why they are ill and indeed to "blame the victim" when his or her inadvisable behavior appears to be the source of the condition.

Health insurance often is priced lower for people who do not smoke and who wear seat belts than for people who use cigarettes and/or don't use seat belts. In a National Institutes of Health consensus conference a few years ago, liver transplants for alcoholics were not recommended because of the high risk of transplant failure. The same recommendation was not made for liver cancer victims, despite the fact that their cancer is about as likely to recur as is cirrhosis.

This attitude makes many people—including me—uncomfortable. I'm not here to defend smoking: I quit it years ago, and I think everyone who smokes should do the same. I also believe that people have some responsibility for taking care of their health.

But I have problems with the victim-blaming philosophy. First, it is applied inconsistently and often serves as a blind for less justifiable attitudes. Second, it violates the basic ethical charge of the care giver.

Take an example I encountered recently. A young man with professional and family responsibilities repeatedly exposed himself to unnecessary health risks. Not only that; he bragged about his ability to withstand this abuse. He jeopardized his own professional future as well as those of people dependent upon him for their success, and eventually it caught up with him. As a consequence of the damage he sustained, he may never work again in his chosen profession. Who is this careless, undeserving, reckless individual? Jim McMahon, the quarterback of the Chicago Bears, sidelined—perhaps permanently—with shoulder injuries.

Mark Siegler, MD, ethics analyst at the University of Chicago, points out that if we're going to blame patients—and deny them care—because we think they brought on their illnesses themselves, then we must be as hard on joggers, skiers, professional athletes (especially boxers and football players), women with anorexia, and workaholics with stress-related diseases as we are on substance abusers, smokers, alcoholics, and the obese.

In fact, we should be even harder on the first group, because research has shown that substance abuse, nicotine addiction, alcoholism, and morbid obesity are related, in part, to genetic factors and can be considered diseases. Overwork, boxing, football, skiing, and the like are strictly voluntary.

Needless to say, this argument does not convince most people: There is a difference, they say, between skiing and heroin addiction. They say skiers don't intend to hurt themselves while addicts do, but research tells us that doing something dangerous and not caring about the consequences can be characteristic of both skiers and addicts.

"Acceptable" vs. "Unacceptable" Abuse

The point is that we make judgments about self-induced disease and injury inconsistently. What I have observed is that self-abuse that is considered "acceptable" tends to reflect the practices and values of middle-class people, who tend to be privately insured for their healthcare. Self-abuse that is considered "unacceptable" tends to be more common among less advantaged (and often publicly insured or uninsured) people whose cultures, practices, and values are foreign to healthcare professionals, whose values tend to be those of the middle and upper layers of society. We simply hold the poor to a different standard.

The other reason that making subjective judgments about patients' "deservingness" is a bad idea is simply that persons who have committed themselves to providing healthcare to people have committed themselves across the board.

It can be very hard on your head to try to figure out whether the person in front of you—who is, regardless of the source of the problem, probably frightened, in pain, and vulnerable—deserves your care or not. It is ethically difficult and emotionally wrenching.

It is much easier to find other means of venting your anger against the reasons for some people hurting themselves. If you want to attack whatever produced the low-income addict, the child-abusing parent, the alcoholic street person, or similarly unattractive patients, you'll need to get mad at a lot more than just the patient. This is appropriate and necessary; but it should not be a war fought at the bedside.

When care givers find themselves frustrated by and angry at what appears to be self-abuse, noncompliance, and irresponsible behavior on the part of patients, they might find it helpful to ask themselves the following questions:

1. **What am I really angry at?** Is the patient alone at fault, or are there other reasons for his or her condition? Am I really angry at this illness, about which I can't do enough—or anything at all? Am I upset with a society that allows this sort of thing to happen? What caused this situation to develop?

2. **Would I be this angry if the patient were my peer?** We all have to wrestle with cultural differences and prejudices (some of them quite understandable); but we need to sort out the differences between being uncomfortable with someone because we don't understand his or her lifestyle and values and being angry at what we believe is socially irresponsible behavior.

3. **Would I be this angry if the patient had a different type of insurance (or had insurance)?** The jokes about "your tax dollars at work" apply to care givers as well; when we think it's *our* money being wasted, we are more judgmental. All I can suggest

in this regard is that you keep those $7,000 military toilet seats in mind.

4.   If this patient had sustained this same illness or injury in a different way, would I feel the same about him or her? If lung cancer patients developed their illness because of smoking, we question their right to healthcare or insurance; if they developed the illness because of exposure to asbestos, we believe them to be victims of injustice. Similarly, if a man contracts AIDS because he had sexual relations with another man, he's guilty; if he contracts it because he had sexual relations with a woman, he's innocent. That's cutting it pretty fine.

5.   Can I vent this anger by seeing to it that others do not end up in a similar plight? There are many ways in which an individual can make a difference in the fights against substance abuse, alcoholism, ignorance of good health habits, high-risk reproductive behavior, child abuse, drunken or drugged driving, and other dangerous behaviors. You might want to make a commitment to fighting one or more of these plagues through prevention.

At some point, care givers who are sick of treating rat bite get the urge to forego the Band-Aids in favor of killing rats. When that finally happens, we can start to address the larger question, which is not an issue of guilt or innocence, but rather one of keeping people from being victimized—by themselves or others—in the first place.

· ·

Ethics by the Numbers

May 1987

Just a historical note: The "AIDS hospital" men-
tioned near the beginning of the article was established
in Texas by AMI, a for-profit hospital firm. It was
closed shortly thereafter because AMI found out what
many people already knew: Most AIDS patients end
up on Medicaid after losing their jobs and insurance,
if they ever had insurance. The hospital, in fact,
became the only for-profit hospital ever to qualify
for membership in the National Association of
Public Hospitals by virtue of its patient case mix
and financial losses.

People in general, and Americans in particular, have a tendency
to compartmentalize. Whether we are making sure that all the
socks are in a certain part of the drawer, or arranging our social relationships so that they don't interfere with work, or making out the
budget, we are given to separating everything in an orderly fashion.

This may be part of our lingering puritan heritage: the sense of
an ordered universe in which there is a grand design to everything.
We even retain proverbs that preached this gospel long ago: "a place
for everything, and everything in its place."

In more recent times we have extended this philosophy to
many of the disciplines and professions we pursue. We distinguish

one profession from another with a complex superstructure of standards, criteria, and educational requirements. We also subdivide those professions, carefully crafting lines of distinction between, say, civil law and criminal law. Social work is not social work: it's clinical, community, or psychiatric social work.

A House Divided

The all-time compartmentalization champs are those of us who work in healthcare. We can probably blame physicians for that. They may have started out as your basic doctors, but today we have pediatric hand surgeons, liver transplant surgeons, and specialists in particular diseases, certain subtypes of those particular diseases, and certain subtypes of those particular diseases that occur in discrete populations, such as an internist who focuses on pneumonia in the elderly.

We organize our healthcare institutions the same way. Acute care and long-term care may live side by side, but they are not intermixed, other than in "swing bed" programs. We have created hospitals for specific diseases ranging from tuberculosis institutions and psychiatric facilities to, most recently, AIDS hospitals.

And hospitals themselves are the soul of compartmentalization: different types of illnesses, different types of treatment, and different patient populations (in the old days, blacks and whites; today, the elderly, women, and children) often are clustered in separate parts of the institution, each in its proper place.

Needless to say, the different duties of the specialized professionals in the specialized sections of the hospital are all discharged through separate channels. Accounting doesn't mix with internal medicine; marketing doesn't spend much time with housekeeping. The hospital becomes a sort of conceptual cable, with many wires all bundled together, but each carrying its own message and occupying its own discrete space.

Healthcare ends up cut into cubes and strings that do not interconnect in a particularly logical fashion. This keeps consultants and human resources professionals busy, and it provides an endless supply of fascinating case studies in organization structure and management.

The old adage may be true: the hospital—and by implication, the multi-provider system—is essentially unmanageable, an assortment of fiefdoms held together by faith, hope, and stubbornness in the face of reality. As someone once observed, "Aerodynamically, the bumble bee shouldn't be able to fly, but the bumble bee doesn't know it, so it goes on flying, anyway."

The Missing Tool

This arrangement may not be all that bad; after all, this is the age of specialization. But it can cause difficulties. One problem is that all this delineation of turf can deny valuable decision-making tools to those people who are trying to make tricky healthcare ethics decisions.

It's a case of parallel development. Today, more and more healthcare policy, payment, and service configuration decisions are being made on the basis of health services research findings. An army of happy analysts working for government, private payers, consulting firms, and employers are unlocking the secrets of the structure and performance of the healthcare system. DRGs, for example, were the product of a health services research project at Yale. Other researchers are now working on ways to refine DRGs to reflect the severity of illness of patients and differences in hospital case-mix.

Some analysts are examining the relationship of the volume of certain procedures performed by a given hospital (or physician) with the quality of the outcomes. The evidence indicates that providers performing a high volume of, say, organ transplants or cholecystectomies seem to have better outcomes (lower mortality, shorter length of stay, fewer complications) than providers performing only a few of these procedures.

One of the oldest and most influential health services research efforts has been analysis of medical practice pattern variations— the fact that different populations, living in areas very near each other, undergo certain healthcare treatments and procedures at wildly different rates.

In Iowa, men in one county have a 15 percent chance of undergoing prostatectomy; men in a nearby county have a 60 percent chance. Hysterectomy rates for women who live to the age of 75 once ranged from 70 percent in one part of Maine to 20 percent in another.

More remarkably, when physicians intervene to question why some rates are as high (or as low) as they are, the rates change. In the town in Maine where the hysterectomy rate was 70 percent, the rate is now much lower, because doctors started talking to each other. The same thing happened with tonsillectomies in Vermont, where the area with the highest rate in the state became a low-rate area after physicians started asking each other why so many tonsillectomies were being done.

Mixing Numbers with Ideas

Logic would dictate that there are profound ethical implications in all this. Does it not raise questions of right and wrong when a hospital is performing more cholecystectomies or cesarean sections than any other hospital in the state? Is there not cause for ethical concern when a medical staff insists on retaining a low-volume service with a mortality rate three times that of other providers that have higher volumes? Yet contact—let alone exchange of information—among practitioners, researchers, and ethics analysts is spotty at best.

This separation of powers is not all that surprising. Ethics, after all, came down a different line in the healthcare cable than research did. For one thing, ethics and philosophy have always been viewed as arts, not sciences; they belong to the liberal arts curriculum and are often seen as being more intellectually pleasant than applicable to the real world.

Medicine, on the other hand, has pushed itself to become a science, forever seeking to be more sure, to find a new way of measuring something, to discover the "magic bullet" of certainty and cure. Physicians may speak of the "art of medicine"—and healthcare certainly does have its philosophical side—but the clinical professions are steeped in science.

Bioethics deliberations take place in the heady atmosphere of the ethics conference, the institutional review board, the institutional ethics committee. Health services research is discussed at scientific meetings and conferences on payment and policy. No wonder there is so little interaction between health services research and ethics.

Yet it seems to me that research, even when it is focused on hard-core issues such as utilization, payment, efficacy, and quality, provides a powerful tool for ethical consideration of healthcare delivery decisions—a tool we are not using.

Not a New Idea

But there are precedents for using this tool. One example—which remains a monument to the courage of those who developed it—is the treatment option program instituted by the burn service of Los Angeles County Medical Center in 1975. Burn center director Bruce Zawacki, MD, and his colleague Sharon Imbus reported on that program in a controversial, landmark article in *The New England Journal of Medicine* in 1977.

What they had done was remarkable. To a greater degree than is the case with many other injuries, burns can be assessed with virtual mathematical precision as to their severity and the chances of a patient surviving them. Even in the Seventies, one could identify patients who had suffered burns of such magnitude that no one had ever been known to survive them.

What the burn professionals on the service did was to inform such "terminally burned" patients, when they were admitted, that no patient anywhere was known to have survived the type of burn they had sustained.

These patients were offered a choice of "heroic," full-blown care or more palliative (and less painful) care that involved suspension of fluid resuscitation, admission to a private room, unlimited visiting hours, and counseling by a nurse, chaplain, and/or others as desired. Of 24 such patients, 21 chose the palliative approach. All 24 died.

That program represented one of the first reported organized efforts to use quantitative research to support patient autonomy—as well as a more humane approach to care when the odds against survival appear insurmountable.

Discussion of such issues is commonplace today; but in 1977, Imbus and Zawacki were attacked in some corners for that article. They were accused of "showboating" and even of abandoning their patients. It is more clear now that they were simply way ahead of the pack in trying to link ethical decision-making with research findings.

How It Might Be Done

I think there ought to be more efforts of this nature, and I would like to suggest a few examples of how such a process could work. They are not as polished as they might be, but they're a start. They might help us at least think about incorporating research into the ethics process. Heaven knows, there is enough muddy, sticky ground in ethics that any objective tool should be welcomed with open arms.

Case No. 1: Should We Offer a Particular Service?

Take coronary artery bypass graft (CABG) surgery as an example. Studies in California and elsewhere have shown that, as a rule, the higher the volume of CABG surgery offered by a hospital, the lower the rate of mortality and other problems resulting from use of that procedure. This is not a hard and fast rule; but it holds in the vast majority of cases.

Now, let's say that a hospital has been offering CABG procedures for a while, but business isn't too good, so only a few dozen a year are being performed. The medical staff or administration learns that the mortality rate among CABG patients at the hospital is much higher than it is at a neighboring hospital that provides hundreds of CABG procedures a year.

Given that a link between volume and mortality has been established, it seems to me that there is an ethical imperative to reassess the hospital's CABG program and, possibly, to consider terminating it if there does seem to be a problem with quality of outcome.

After all, ethics is the study of doing the right thing; it seems to me that harming patients through the ill-advised continuation of a risky service is incompatible with appropriate ethical behavior.

Similarly, many hospitals are considering heart transplant programs, either because they wish to provide this service to their constituents or because all the publicity around the procedure might give the hospital a marketing edge. In their deliberations, these hospitals should keep firmly in mind the fact that the supply of donor hearts in the United States—no matter how we try to increase donations—will never come close to meeting demand. Furthermore, a link between heart transplant center volume and better outcomes has also been established.

If these research findings are not incorporated into the examination of the ethics of opening a transplant center, the hospital is missing the boat. The hospital will not benefit anyone (including itself) if it offers a low-volume program that produces poor outcomes and squanders precious donor organs.

Case No. 2: How Can We Best Serve the Medically Indigent?

A hospital has a mission to serve the medically indigent, but it has limited resources to devote to that mission. Up until now, it has taken all comers in its emergency department, thereby focusing its indigent care dollars on whomever comes into that department *in extremis*.

Research into the matter shows that the most common service requested is obstetrics—and that the medically indigent women whose infants are delivered at the hospital are far more likely than insured women to have received little or no prenatal care and to lose their babies at birth.

A little more research will yield the infant mortality rate in the community, as well as the extent of medical indigence among women of child-bearing age. These statistics could help the hospital stretch those obstetrics dollars by trying to reach these women early in their pregnancies with prenatal care and other help, such as information about nutrition programs.

If it is not in conflict with the hospital's mission and values, information about family planning might also be offered to medically indigent women who are at risk of unwanted pregnancy. This will quite likely lead to lower obstetrics costs, fewer high-risk mothers, and lower infant mortality.

This is not a hypothetical case; more than a few hospitals are trying to use health status and demographic research in this way. A major program was just inaugurated in Chicago whereby community hospitals in neighborhoods with high infant mortality rates will be working with public health authorities to intervene earlier in potentially high-risk pregnancies.

Case No. 3: Are We Putting Patients at Risk?

Let's say that Community Hospital has a very successful cesarean section program, providing large numbers of the procedure every year. In the next town, Memorial Hospital provides very few cesarean sections. An analysis of the practice pattern variations in the area shows that while Community's cesarean section rate is three times that of the state average, Memorial's rate is the lowest in the state. (There are currently many states where cesarean section rates do, in fact, fall into this sort of pattern.) Is there an ethics issue here?

Could be. It is possible that Community is not conservative enough about cesarean section—after all, it is often a profitable procedure, and many physicians believe it protects them against malpractice litigation. It could also be that Memorial is too unwilling to provide them. *Or it could be both*. It would behoove the institutional ethics committees or ethics analysts at both institutions to ask the medical staff to look at these variations and try to find out why they exist.

There are two major issues here. One is the first Hippocratic dictum: The healthcare provider should do no harm. Are patients receiving risky surgery when they don't need it, because the procedure is profitable? Or are patients being denied a procedure that could benefit them and their babies simply because the hospital's HMO and PPO contracts make it more profitable to restrict the availability of cesarean sections?

Neither situation sounds like a very moral way to run a railroad. And yet data are available, and have been for years, that can help show when cesarean section is indicated, when it is not, the advantages of normal delivery, the feasibility of trial labor, and the risks of cesareans.

Many public figures are announcing that the "rationing" of healthcare is inevitable—that the availability of beneficial services will have to be restricted. If that is true (and I have my doubts, but that's another column), it becomes incumbent upon the healthcare system to use its resources in the most responsible and efficient way possible.

Denying beneficial care to patients should hardly be done lightly. It should be the very last of last resorts and should be postponed until absolutely no other option is available. Therefore, *ethical principles require responsible use of resources*. And health services research provides information that can be used to "flag" wasteful practices and identify potential areas of concern in terms of over-care and under-care alike.

In a nation that spends more money per capita than any other on healthcare and still ranks seventeenth in the world in infant mortality, a stronger ethical stance on use of resources, backed up by reliable research, would seem to be very much in order.

The Ethics of Curiosity

It is possible that after considering the ethics of these or similar situations, the leaders of a hospital, HMO, group practice, or health-care system might decide that they want to go ahead with what appears to be ethically contraindicated. They might do so for reasons related to market position, public image, or revenue enhancement. That is their choice.

But any choice should be made with full knowledge of the situation and of the options available. Not to tap the ever-growing pool of health services research information as part of such a process seems foolhardy.

It is not difficult to find out what's happening in health services research. The annual meetings of the American Public Health Association and the Association for Health Services Research are laced with presentations by major researchers. JAMA (the *Journal of the American Medical Association*), the *New England Journal of Medicine*, *Medical Care*, *Health Affairs*, *Health Services Research*, and the *Medicine and Health* and *Utilization Management* newsletters from Faulkner and Gray, among others, offer a wealth of research information.

Many of the researchers who work in these centers would be pleased to attend a hospital ethics committee session, ethics conference, or medical staff meeting to discuss what health services research is teaching us—and how we can use it in ethical decision-making.

William Foege, MD, outgoing president of the American Public Health Association, in his 1986 presidential address, quoted a writer named Larry Levinger: "All over America, we are struggling to know, is a Honda better than a Volkswagen? Can computers sell cows? Does Saturn have air? Do prunes cause diabetes? Will magnetism heal bones? We want to know how to bake righteous muffins and grow back hair. We are just a curious people, poking around the house, reading the Corn Flakes label and answering the phone."

This marvelous curiosity has spawned a health services research community that is finding out more and more about how health-care works—and how it *should* work. Our need to know has also produced an ethics community whose members have beaten their heads against the walls of intractable dilemmas for thousands of years, seeking that most elusive prize: the right thing to do. It seems to me, in these latter and more enlightened days, that it's about time these two communities—linked as they are in parallel and potentially mutually supportive quests—start talking to each other.

Ethics Down Under

Same Songs, Different Tunes

July 1987

This was the product of a visit to Australia to have a look at its healthcare system. The grand controversy over in vitro fertilization and surrogate motherhood has died down to the barest of whispers in both that nation and this one, but many of the nursing issues I encountered there are still very much part of health-care life in the United States.

It's extraordinarily valuable to learn how another culture is con-fronting healthcare ethics issues. However, there's always the ques-tion of whether what they're doing is applicable to what we're doing.

I recently returned from Australia, where I learned something about the healthcare system and spent some time visiting with bioethicists. I was curious as to whether ethics Down Under would have any parallels with what we're pondering up here.

I needn't have wondered. At least two of the issues drawing the attention of healthcare practitioners and ethics analysts in Australia are eerily familiar to American healthcare professionals: artificial (or least unusual) means of fertilization and the future of nursing.

These were among the chief issues I discussed with bioethicists Peter Singer, director of the Centre for Human Bioethics at Monash University in Melbourne, and his colleagues, codirector Helga Kuhse, researcher Karen Dawson, and attorney Pascal Kasimba, as

well as Nick Tonti-Filippini, director of bioethics at St. Vincent's
Hospital in Melbourne.

Much Ado About Nothing?

In vitro fertilization (IVF) has become a major concern in Australia
during the past few years, partially because the technology was
developed there (Louise Brown, the first child produced through an
IVF procedure, was born in Australia). Programs are continuing,
despite a rather low (17–20 percent) success rate.

Ethics questions raised by IVF include the social and moral
acceptability of the procedure itself, the fate of fertilized embryos
that are not implanted, research use of embryos, and the occasionally raised issue of the amount of healthcare resources that should
be devoted to what critics see as an exotic and often unsuccessful
procedure. Because of these concerns, as well as the intense public
attention it has received, says Professor Singer, IVF "has greatly
enhanced public awareness and discussion of ethical issues."

One cannot help but note the similarities between this debate in
a nation 13,000 miles away from our own, and the recent furor in our
country over surrogate motherhood. Indeed, the massive publicity
and controversy engendered by the Stern-Whitehead child custody
battle in the New Jersey "Baby M" case was due almost exclusively to
differences of opinion over various aspects of surrogate motherhood.

In both cases, massive press coverage, proclamations in publica-
tions and broadcasts, international attention, and the deliberations
of many skilled ethical minds are all focusing on a procedure that is
unlikely to touch more than a tiny fraction of the population.

What is it that makes IVF or surrogacy so compelling, when
there are other issues that scream for attention—issues that affect
far more people? Australia is trying to decide the extent of healthcare coverage the population should have under its universal entitlement. The United States is in the shameful position of ranking
eighteenth in the world and last among developed nations in terms

of our infant mortality rate (10.8 deaths per 1,000 births in 1984, the last year for which data are available). Yet both countries are obsessed with the ethics of some forms of artificial insemination.

I suspect that the reasons for this apparently lopsided sense of priorities are different in the two countries. Australia is, after all, an island—albeit a large one—that is half a world away from other Anglo-Celtic, English-speaking cultures. IVF is perhaps its best known home-grown healthcare technology, and it is therefore not surprising that IVF has become a lightning rod for the development of bioethics consciousness and discussion.

In the United States, motherhood is usually a compelling subject, within and outside of healthcare. We also have an almost unnatural preoccupation with lurid or emotional legal cases (what I call the Perry Mason Syndrome). The "Baby M" case was made to order for national overemphasis.

Is all the attention appropriate? Well, in Australia, IVF has served a valuable purpose in sparking awareness of bioethics, and study of the issues surrounding this and related forms of insemination will undoubtedly educate us all. But I have to be something of a spoilsport about the surrogacy issue in the United States.

Despite all the drama and tears and intense press coverage, surrogacy will never touch more than one one-thousandth of one percent of American lives. I'd much rather see more attention paid to our horrifying infant mortality rate and to the extremely difficult issues faced daily by caregivers in hospitals with regard to very sick and severely disabled newborns and infants.

The Nursing Shortage—An Ethical Issue

The other issue that the Australian ethicists raised also has a direct parallel in American healthcare. It was a little spooky for me to read the American Hospital Association report on the nursing shortage (83 percent of American hospitals with nursing vacancies, declining enrollment in nursing schools, a lessening of interest in the profession among high school and college students) and then go halfway around the world, only to have Australian ethics analysts cite nursing as the most critical healthcare issue in their country.

Nick Tonti-Filippini says that "the changing role of the nurse is gradually overwhelming all other issues" of moral discussion in Australia. Kuhse says that "problems with nursing in Australia appear to be economic," but are based on much deeper social problems. Everyone cited a long 1986 strike by nurses in the state of Victoria as having brought the issue to the fore.

Many nurses in Australia feel "a total dissatisfaction" with the profession, according to Kuhse. They are increasingly restless with their traditional role of "physician extender" as they become more prideful and sophisticated as a profession. Tonti-Filippini believes that the relationship of nurses to physicians needs redefinition and that the process of reshaping that definition is likely to be difficult for all involved.

Sounded very *deja vu* to me. American healthcare providers are slowly coming to face the fact that nursing now must compete for the attention of young women with many other professions (including medicine), not just with teaching. And 96 percent of nurses are still women. Certainly part of the underlying disadvantage faced by nursing in such a competition is that although it has the sublime appeal of being a caring profession with a proud heritage and a strong sense of honor, its practitioners often have to run a gamut of physicians, administrators, and boards who think nurses either are doormats or should be.

Bioethics and the Future of Nursing

What does that have to do with ethics? Why do these Australian ethics analysts see the redefinition of nursing as a moral issue? I can see two ways in which the future of nursing is central to bioethics.

First, no matter how an institution or system approaches its ethics dilemmas, and no matter what process it sets up, the success or failure of its activities will be determined by the participation, support and enthusiasm of its nursing staff—or the lack thereof. Nurses already have figured prominently in key ethics discussions—from the *Barber* case, in which physicians were accused of murder for terminating life support, to the recent George Washington University study that found that more autonomy for ICU nurses may improve the chances of survival of very sick ICU patients. I think evidence is building toward the conclusion that much of the quality of ethical decision-making and education will be determined by nurses. It is nurses, after all, who must live with, and often must carry out, the results of the institutional ethics process.

Second, it's difficult to have great nursing staff participation in the ethics process if you don't have many nurses. In fact, it's difficult to keep the place going if you don't have enough nurses. Well, the nursing shortage did not arrive on a moonbeam. It is partially the result of the fact that too many nurses believe they have gotten something of a raw deal. They have been saddled with the double vulnerability of being women and of being seen as a sort of clinical second fiddle.

The ethics issue here is the level of respect employers accord to employees—and whether it is morally justifiable to treat a critically important profession like dirt for decades, just because you could get away with it. This has to do with the ethics of management, which are no less important than the ethics of patient autonomy or end-of-life decisions.

I don't know where the road will end, either for IVF or for nursing. The Catholic Church statement condemning IVF was issued while I was in Australia, and Singer was scheduled to debate Tonti-Filippini on the subject right after I left Melbourne. Shortly after I came home, the "Baby M" case was settled—and the decision appealed. Both Australia and the US face a revolt against the traditional roles relegated to nurses by the healthcare system. The beat goes on. But it's reassuring, in a misery-loves-company sort of way, to know that we're not alone.

Buying into the Doctor's Decision

More Than We Bargained For?

September 1987

Physics tells us that, for the most part, any reaction that proceeds one way can reverse itself and go back the other way. This principle can provide a pretty useful world view, especially because it reassures us that the tide of human affairs rarely flows in only one direction.

However, there are times in the current healthcare world when one wonders if the laws of physics (and of everything else) are in the process of being broken. And nowhere is that possibility more real than in the changing relationship between physicians and patients.

Embedded in the growing militancy and consumer-oriented attitudes of patients is a serious question of ethics: Have the changes in the physician-patient relationship created a situation that is irreversible, but should not be? In seeking a greater, even dominant, role in healthcare decision-making, have patients bitten off more than they can chew?

Certainly, things have changed. In the old days—from the reign of the Romans until about 15 years ago—we entrusted physicians with most of our major healthcare decisions. The doctor told us what to do, or what had happened, and we believed him or her. It was a classic trust relationship, imbued with all the advantages and threats one-sided trust relationships can have.

That relationship developed because people needed a way to deal with one of the essential inequities in healthcare delivery: the fact that providers hold a monopoly on information. Put simply, healers have traditionally known things the rest of us did not know.

Women, Wizardry, and Healing

It has not even mattered who the healers are. In many societies, the folkloric power of women (probably attributed to them because of the magical nature of gestation, childbirth, and the renewal of life they represent) led them to be the healers. In some societies, they still are.

Any person, male or female, who could make other people well was assumed to have special gifts. This elevated the healer to a spiritual level that undoubtedly made her or his work easier because part of healing is trust and belief on the part of the patient.

This may have been all hocus-pocus, but if the patient believed the healer knew what he or she was doing, it enhanced the healing process. I think this simple fact was known long before the behavioral psychologists proved it with research.

Equating healing with magic contributed to the healers' information monopoly: A successful healer knew how to save lives or to improve health while other people did not. If you believe a person has superior skill because of magic, you can accept the hoarding of critical information.

If you believe that *anyone* can have healing skills, and that healers are just withholding information in order to increase their income, prestige, or power, then conflict is guaranteed. The trust relationship between healer and patient is shattered. And as a result, the healing process suffers a setback.

Lost Faith

This relationship between healer and patient lasted for a very long time, but in recent years it has started to unravel. There are many reasons for this, including increasing consumer awareness, the collision of the women's movement with medicine, the *Quinlan* case, the coming of treatments that can prevent death but don't exactly produce a sterling quality of life, and the *perceived* arrogance and insensitivity of medical practitioners. And the fact that physicians make so much money doesn't exactly stem the tide of resentment either.

Patients today are much less willing to accept what a doctor says as the last word; they are more interested in participating in all the decisions affecting their healthcare. Most of us who lean toward a libertarian view of life can hardly quarrel with such a trend.

I, for one, would find it unthinkable to undergo nonemergency surgery without a second opinion, or to agree to a unilateral decision made by a physician about what should—or should not—be done for a terminally ill friend or relative. Nevertheless, when we decide to buy into the doctor's decision-making process, we may get more than we bargain for.

In his book, *Hard Choices* (G.P. Putnam & Sons, New York City, 1986), B.D. Colen, science editor of *Newsday*, explores the issue of anencephalic infants—children born without a cerebral cortex—who, in his words, "have no self-awareness, let alone an ability to receive and return love." Colen observes that Cara Lynn, the child he discusses as an example, was, "from the moment of her birth, a candidate for infanticide."

He points out that it has long been common practice, when a terribly malformed infant is born, to place the child face down in a tray in the delivery room, where it will shortly die. The parents are informed that the child was stillborn.

Few anencephalic children survive, with or without care. But Cara Lynn did, and her parents have been burdened with the inordinate human, social, and financial cost of caring constantly for a child who does not know that they are there—or that she is there, for that matter. Under the circumstances, it is no wonder that a physician Colen interviewed said that in letting Cara Lynn live, some physician "didn't do his job."

Who Decides?

The question, of course, is whether unilateral decision-making in such situations is still the physician's job. Many other parties—including other physicians, nurses, attorneys, political figures, patients, families, and journalists—now want part of the action when the case involves issues of treatment or nontreatment, life support versus termination of support, intervention or letting nature take its course. The doctor does not have sole proprietorship over such decision-making anymore.

This may be as it should be. However, in disrupting the physician's private decision-making process, the rest of us have done more than merely join that process. We have permanently altered the range of options, for there are certain decisions that can only be made by one person, in private.

Just look at the situation of Cara Lynn and other anencephalic newborns. If you consult with others about whether you should abandon such a life, you give up your right to decide in secret.

The decision, at that point, becomes a *matter of record*. And in the US, once behavior becomes a matter of record, that behavior tends to change. We behave differently in our social and public lives than in our individual, private lives. Just ask Richard Nixon or Gary Hart.

Does this mean that, in these truly awful, no-win situations, we should hand the decision-making back to physicians, and move the entire process back into the closet? Of course not. Even if we wanted to do so, it's not possible to turn back the clock. Unlike the laws of physics, in this situation reversal is not possible.

The governing principle here is illustrated by the myth of "Pandora's Box": Once the critter gets out, you can't coax it back into its container. Knowing what we now know, it is highly unlikely that we could ever talk ourselves into once again accepting physicians' decisions without question.

Furthermore, it's not fair to physicians to still expect them to be magicians. As long as we accepted magical powers and spiritual superiority as part of the healer's characteristics, we could accept with equal faith the idea that the healer was also always right. If a physician was omnipotent, he or she was also omniscient. We would not be mired in the current disastrous malpractice situation if we still believed that. Doctors make mistakes, just like everybody else, thought it's a little different when they mess up, because the stakes are much higher.

Punishing Physicians

The problem is that we don't want to allow the possibility of mistakes by our healers, so we punish physicians in every possible way when they do commit errors. We fail to differentiate between mistakes that could have been reasonably avoided and occurrences that were inevitable and for which blame should not be assessed.

It turns out that our consumerism and militancy are still draped with shreds of old beliefs. The fact that physicians fail to live up to ancient and outmoded expectations is one reason we challenge them. But if we now say that physicians cannot have hegemony over us without being questioned, we should tell ourselves the same thing. We cannot demand to be part of physician decision-making and yet continue to believe in doctors' inherent magic.

Decisions such as termination of treatment, nonresuscitation, nontreatment of the terribly distressed or malformed, and discontinuation or nonimplementation of life support are just too damned difficult to lay on one person, no matter how well trained or prepared that individual is to make such choices.

These options are better explored through collaboration, discussion, sharing of ideas, examination of prior experience, and debate of what is best for whom. That's why I support institutional ethics committees, ethics consultations, and the commitment by healthcare organizations to raise the consciousness of their employees and professional staff concerning ethics issues and problems.

As we have taken away the physician's magic wand and invincible armor, we must join him or her in horrid, wrenching decisions as well as in more clear-cut, satisfying ones. We must offer physicians support just as we seek it from them. We've jumped out of the frying pan of uninformed acceptance of doctors' decisions, and have landed in the fire of trying to make those decisions ourselves.

AIDS and Insurers

Keeping the Covenant?

November 1987

See the headnote for "Of Providers and Plagues"
(page 14).

Health insurance was set up to cover unpredictable events—and AIDS is no longer an unpredictable event." This observation from a noted economist at a recent national meeting came as a response to concerns voiced by Peter Arno, assistant professor of healthcare administration at Mount Sinai School of Medicine in New York City. He fears a virtual total loss of private health insurance by Americans with AIDS—precisely because a person's chances of developing AIDS can be predicted through antibody testing.

Arno's worries appear to be well-founded. According to a report in the July 16, 1987, *New England Journal of Medicine*, "Approximately half of all insurance companies use AIDS-antibody tests for *individual* health and life policies." The practice is barred only in California and the District of Columbia, as of this writing. (Wisconsin implemented a similar law and then withdrew it.)

But the vast majority of people with health insurance are members of employee groups and insurers do not require testing of group members. The problem is that health insurance is usually employment-based. If you lose your job, you lose your insurance.

If you have AIDS or AIDS-related complex (ARC), the odds are that sooner or later you will have to quit work. You may then try to obtain individual insurance—and be required to take an HIV antibody test. But at that point, you will not need to worry about testing because AIDS is a pre-existing condition that will not be covered by most insurance policies anyway.

A Public Sector Disease

A great many AIDS and ARC patients are not insured to begin with. Most homosexual Americans are employed and many are insured, but many low-income immigrants and most intravenous drug abusers and prostitutes are not working in insured jobs. Their only choices are Medicaid or indigence.

Medicaid is already showing the strain. The Rand Corporation has estimated that of the $37 billion that AIDS treatment could cost in 1991, Medicaid may shell out $10 billion. A recent study of AIDS costs by the National Association of Public Hospitals (NAPH) provides grim evidence of the shift of AIDS to public sponsorship.

Of the AIDS patients treated in 49 public hospitals in 1985, says Dennis Andrulis, director of policy and research for NAPH, 92 percent were paid for by some form of public funding: Medicare sponsored 1.3 percent of them, prison health systems covered 4.1 percent, and Medicaid covered a whopping 61.8 percent. Another 25.2 percent were "self-pay," which usually means "no pay." Private insurance covered only 7.7 percent.

Even more distressing was the disproportionately lower amount of Medicaid funding for AIDS patients in the South as opposed to other areas of the US (see table). Disenfranchisement of AIDS patients from private coverage is not a possibility; for public hospital patients, it is a reality.

Medicaid might eventually play an even larger role as more AIDS patients live long enough to survive the two-year waiting period and qualify for the program by reason of disability. Federal authorities have risen to this challenge with a shoddy game of sleight-of-hand.

Funding of AIDS Patients in 49 Public Hospitals in 1985 According to Geographic Area (%)

	Medicaid (%)	Private Insurance (%)	"Self-Pay" (%)
Northeast	68	6.1	18.3
West	60.3	11.2	26.3
Midwest	57	23.4	13
South	16.4	6.0	73.6

A new low was reached when the Reagan Administration proposed that Medicare stop reimbursing hospitals for bad debts of Medicare clients who do not pay deductibles and co-payments—and that the money thus saved be used for AIDS research and education! It seems obvious that Medicare is not going to leap at the chance to insure AIDS patients—unless someone else is disenfranchised to pay for it.

One of the greatest ironies of AIDS is that AMI's proprietary Institute for Immunological Disorders, the Houston hospital opened specifically to care for AIDS patients, suffered losses so enormous that it became the first for-profit hospital ever to qualify for membership in NAPH. After a reported $5 million in uncompensated care losses, AMI announced last August that the hospital would be closed.

"A Private Sector Contractual Relationship"

Not all private insurers have bailed out on the AIDS population. Blue Cross and Blue Shield plans still treat AIDS like any other disease. The Maryland Blues, in fact, have developed a model policy that may be duplicated elsewhere. Their policy, not requiring testing of existing or new policyholders, also prohibits discrimination against employees with AIDS.

The question remains: Are the insurers who do pick and choose justified? Richard Schweiker, president of the American Council of

Life Insurance, has been quoted as saying, "Insurance is, after all, not a public social system but a private-sector contractual relationship." If that is so, then it is just good business to cut losses, skim the good risks, and avoid those in desperate need.

But it is just not that simple. In the first place, insurance—especially health insurance—is not *only* "a private-sector contractual relationship." Americans see it as something broader, which is why we regulate it, monitor it, mandate benefits, and surround it with many of the trappings of a social program (including significant tax advantages for its purchasers).

Also, many "private-sector contractual relationships" fall into the sphere of social accountability; the physician/patient relationship and the hospital/patient relationship come to mind. These are among the most private of contracts; but they are also recognized as having broad social implications.

Providers are expected to protect their patients and information about them, to offer care to those who cannot pay, to uphold high moral standards. Providers get clobbered if they don't do these things. The same should hold for health insurers, who enjoy the benefits of special social status but don't seem to feel accountable.

The private insurance industry has offered a solution for the problem of AIDS coverage. It supports state risk pools for the "uninsurable." Unfortunately, states with such pools have learned that most chronically ill or otherwise uninsurable individuals also cannot afford the high premiums these pools must charge in order to achieve solvency. And the pools aren't solvent; they require subsidy.

As a result, Arno says, fewer than 21,000 people are enrolled in state pools—of an estimated 37 million medically indigent Americans.

What is needed is a *real* "public/private partnership," not the jettisoning of HIV-positive individuals and ARC and AIDS sufferers into public programs alone. Private insurers must take on some of the responsibility.

I understand that this is going to cost. Indeed, Carl Schramm, president of the Health Insurance Association of America, has said that if private insurers are to participate more in coverage of AIDS, the cost of everyone's premiums will go up.

So what else is new? That often happens when the cost of healthcare goes up, or new technology is introduced, or a new illness or condition raises its ugly head. I thought health insurance was based on the principle that a lot of folks toss some money into a common pot from which each can draw if he or she needs it.

Each individual will need more or less of it, at different times, so the disbursement is not equal. But no one expects it to be. That's why it's a communal exercise. The idea goes back to the old funeral societies, from which modern insurance draws much of its heritage and philosophy.

It Is Not My Problem

There are those, too, who say that AIDS is not a universal threat, and therefore, although the insurance situation is unfortunate, it's not their problem. And let's face it: Although AIDS treads a broader path today than it did when it was known as the "gay disease," it is not yet a general epidemic.

Its effect on the population as a whole has been much less catastrophic than the toll it has taken among those most vulnerable to it, therefore many folks do not think that the collapse of insurance for this illness has to do with them. If you are one of these people, let me offer reasons why you should think again.

Even if you do not see the uninsurability of AIDS as a personal threat, you should understand that it represents a dire threat to healthcare providers. For if private coverage disappears, all of that $37 billion must come out of public pockets.

Currently, 75 percent of Medicaid expenditures are being consumed by care of the elderly, blind, and disabled—chiefly for long-term care. If most AIDS funding must come from that embattled program, you can bet that it will be carved out of someone else's hide—like healthcare providers or AFDC (aid to Families with Dependent Children) mothers and children.

Furthermore, most middle-class, monogamous, non-drug-using Americans may not be at great risk of AIDS, but we are all at great risk of *something*. If we allow insurers to disenfranchise by diagnosis, it will be our turn one of these days. AIDS is simply the first major illness on a long, long road. At the end of that road will be a world in which no one who needs health insurance can get it, while the needs of the sick and potentially sick overwhelm limited public health resources.

Well, everything has a silver lining, they say. Those of us who worry about medical indigence know that down that road also lies universal health coverage. And if we keep on the way we are going, unmet need will become so overwhelming that the US will enact a universal entitlement, as most other developed nations have done.

Keeping the Covenant

At the core of the fight over AIDS and insurance is a threat to a basic ethic: What is our responsibility to ourselves as a society? In his elegantly philosophical murder novel, *A Covenant with Death*, Stephen Becker suggests that the reason we gathered together as societies was that people struck a deal with each other. The agreed-upon covenant was, "I will be one of you, if you will protect me." Hence, says Becker, as long as the group affords protection and shared resources, the individual agrees not to bust up the place— and is rightly punished if he or she breaks that agreement.

We cannot live in today's world without such a covenant. In being part of society, even on a shallow level, we agree to trust each other to some degree. Think about it the next time you are driving. Imagine what traffic would be like if we all decided that we need not watch out for the other guy or follow the rules.

Whatever definitions insurers choose for themselves, the fact is that the public sees insurance as a means of common, mutual protection—an expression of the old covenant. Excluding AIDS patients from that bond jeopardizes the very existence of that covenant. If we allow the rules to be broken in this one instance, breaking them will be that much easier. As the saying goes in England, "If the pie's already cut, who's going to mind another slice?"

I maintain that coverage against the vagaries of ill health is, or should be, a type of common possession, something we all need and should have. Sometimes self-expression is most forcefully achieved through reinforcing one's alliance with the group—restating one's relationship to the rest of humanity. Fighting the isolation, disenfranchisement, and abandonment of AIDS patients by insurers would be an excellent place to start.

When Everyone Is Right

January 1988

Recently, Vermont folklorist Margaret MacArthur told me the legend of Duncan Campbell, lord of Inverawe Castle in Scotland. One night a stranger, covered with blood, knocked at the lord's door and asked for shelter. The stranger said he had just killed someone and made Campbell swear to protect him.

Soon other men arrived, seeking the stranger—who had killed Campbell's cousin. Though aghast, Campbell still feigned ignorance of the man's whereabouts, honoring the oath he had made. That night, his cousin's ghost appeared to him and warned him not to hide the murderer. Campbell took the killer out of his house and hid him in a cave, trying to honor both his oath and his family allegiance. Again the ghost appeared, prophesying that Campbell would suffer for protecting the stranger: Campbell and his son, members of the Black Watch regiment, were killed in the battle of Ticonderoga in 1758.

Campbell's dilemma may sound familiar to caregivers who are often caught between two claims of right or two conflicting duties. A patient's family begs a nurse not to tell the patient that he or she is dying because they believe the patient will become morbidly depressed or even suicidal. The nurse agrees. Then the patient asks if he or she is dying. What does the nurse do?

An administrator or trustee is torn between upholding the provider's mission to serve the poor and a desire to keep the organization financially solvent. He or she says that patients who cannot pay must be turned away, honoring one organizational mission while compromising another.

There is no neat way to resolve these value conflicts, but I can suggest some guidelines for doing so.

- **Identify organizational, professional, or personal traps.** If the hospital board promulgates a completely unrealistic mission statement, challenge it. If the marketing department launches a misleading advertising campaign, question it. If physicians are making unrealistic promises to patients, confront those physicians. Otherwise you—or the line nurse, administrator, clerk, or housekeeper—may end up knee-deep in moral conflict.

- **Seek the advice of others.** In a deep moral crisis—such as that experienced by a nurse when she or he believes that a very popular physician is endangering a patient—the tendency is to try to work it out alone. Although confidentiality must be guarded, there is usually *someone* to consult—an ethics counselor or ethics committee member, clergyman, employee assistance program staff member, your personal physician or attorney. Don't "tough it out" alone.

- **Decide who or what should be served first.** The best way to come to an ethical solution is to decide which interests have priority. This can do wonders to clarify one's thinking. Priorities to consider are the patient, the family, religious beliefs, professional honor, personal values, the good of the organization, and the good of society.

- **Don't make promises you can't keep.** In the effort to make things easy for patients it often seems better to tell them what they seem to want to hear—this takes less time and provokes fewer questions. Such supposed kindness will come back to haunt you because in the guise of easing pain, you engage in deception. Don't be set up by lying, ignoring the obvious, or agreeing to serve two conflicting masters. Had Duncan Campbell asked some questions when the stranger demanded protection, he would not have ended up in such a bind.

• **Understand that there is no magic bullet.** Examine the problem and make a decision with an eye toward the *optimal* solution, not necessarily the *perfect* solution.

The ethical decision-making process in healthcare is laced with inexactitude, and everyone involved in it makes difficult—and sometimes wrong—choices. Whatever the results, if you pursued an honorable process and did your best, do not punish yourself: Many people have had to make horrible, "lifeboat" decisions.

If there is any wheel that does not need to be reinvented, it is the agony of learning how to make tough ethical decisions. Formally or informally, share what you have learned in going through an ordeal so someone else's suffering will be diminished. Eventually, we may accumulate enough knowledge and wisdom so that situations of conflicting rights will not be so devastating. The important thing is to have the courage to decide, the intelligence to learn from the experience, and the will to move on.

The Essential Element

May 1988

Certain ethical issues are so difficult to resolve that they keep haunting us—they are the moral equivalents of bad pennies. One of healthcare's most persistent ethical dilemmas is the question of how to define a common foundation of care, or "essential healthcare services."

We keep trying to delineate those services that are "essential" for everyone: Medicare and Medicaid puzzle over what services to cover; private payers try to wait until a procedure—such as an organ transplant—is no longer experimental before they will pay for it. Quality review (what little there is that is not a blind for compulsive cost containment) also seeks to define the essential. Not surprisingly, when the definition of "essential" is established, it turns out to be a narrow one indeed—look at Medicaid's sometimes outrageously stringent definitions of necessary care.

When people start to talk about defining or limiting something, too often they are doing so because they want to establish a ceiling, not a foundation. Although many of the calls for guaranteed access to "essential" services are sincere attempts to ensure that people in need will not go without, frequently they result in placing healthcare services beyond the reach of prospective, often vulnerable patients: the poor, the elderly, the newborn, the very ill.

This issue, therefore, is ethically perilous. What is essential for one person is irrelevant or could be damaging to another. When

most people speak of "essential healthcare services," they are referring to immunization, prenatal and delivery care, and therapy for
treatable cancers—services that we know can produce good outcomes for many, many patients.

But what constitutes essential care to the parents of a child who
is dying of liver disease? One liver transplant? Two? Ten? When
Ronnie DeSillers died in 1987 after a succession of three liver transplants, his parents had been in the process of seeking a fourth liver
for him. That fourth attempt was as important to them as the first.

At the other end of the spectrum are parents whose religious or
social beliefs lead them to eschew immunization of their offspring
against dangerous childhood diseases. To these parents, what most
of us think of as essential is not necessary.

Another reason for ethical concern is that defining what is
absolutely necessary (or essential) presupposes that we know what
works and what does not. Would that medicine were so exact! (Jonas
Salk recently remarked on the polio vaccine he developed: He
didn't know *how* it worked, only that it worked.) No dread disease—
with the possible exception of AIDS—is 100 percent fatal; a few
patients always beat the odds—or die unexpectedly.

It is an ethical imperative that research and data be used whenever possible to determine if care is needed and is worth the risk.
But in many instances, pertinent research has not yet been done
and data are not available to dispel uncertainty. Without such
guideposts, we cannot always know what will or will not work in a
given situation. Thus, clinical uncertainty makes the search for
"essential" services an exercise in ethical shadowboxing.

Although I applaud the sincere efforts to rationalize the basis of
healthcare, I continue to view the search for this new "Holy Grail"
with some skepticism. Nevertheless, I would like to offer the
searchers some advice.

I believe that three criteria are critical in defining "essential"
healthcare. First, those services that *demonstrably* benefit the largest
numbers of people at a reasonable cost should be favored—an idea

in keeping with life in a democracy. For example, I would give immunization and prenatal care higher priority than pancreas transplants. Second, priorities must be set on the basis of *need* and *experience*, rather than on the basis of profitability.

Third, the reason for defining what constitutes "essential" care must be valid, not based upon a desire to reduce vulnerable people's access to healthcare. For as long as there is an inverse relationship between the availability of healthcare and people's need for it, the process of defining essential types of care will be hazardous. There will always be disputes about the necessity of one service over another, but there should be agreement on what is the most essential element of all in the definition process: justice.

Leading Us On

July 1988

There is a well-known joke about Viscount Horatio Nelson, England's greatest naval hero and victor over the Napoleonic fleet at Trafalgar on October 21, 1805. Nelson, it is said, always called for his red coat at the beginning of a battle. He believed that if he was injured during combat, the red coat would hide the blood and thus prevent his men from being demoralized by his injury. The joke concerns the time Nelson's fleet was surrounded by a huge enemy force, all the ships of which were about to fire upon him at point-blank range. Grasping the situation, the viscount called for his brown trousers.

This joke has something to teach us about healthcare leadership in competitive times. When examples of great leadership are sought, military men (and, occasionally, women) are often cited. Given the many parallels between combat and the marketplace, military leaders can probably teach us a lot; indeed, as healthcare providers fight over the shrinking number of insured patients, the lessons of combat seem highly relevant.

That causes me some concern. For one thing, combat requires leadership *against* something or someone. Unity is sought in the face of a common enemy. I shudder to think that an alliance against all comers may serve as the basis for leadership in healthcare.

When I think of leadership, I think of consensus-building, risk-taking, and questioning of the status quo—actions that are undesirable in combat. Furthermore, morality is too often optional in the heat of battle, as the bloody litany of unnecessary slaughter down through the ages illustrates.

So I fear the "combat mentality" that is taking over in many healthcare executive suites and board rooms. Although healthcare's competitive marketplace is being driven by regulation and under-payment as much as by some vague ideological commitment to competition, the fact is that many providers believe they are at war with their peers. In such times, the leader who seeks to discharge his or her responsibilities within a moral framework may be seen as a wimp, a loser, or "not aggressive enough."

We are thus treated to the spectacle of hospitals racing to dupli-cate services already widely available—despite evidence that low-volume, high-technology services often have high mortality rates. We see uninsured patients shuttled back and forth between hospi-tals like so much unwanted refuse. Plots are hatched to swipe key physicians or nurses from the hospital down the street. Healthcare executives whisper innuendos about their peers, and advertising campaigns intimate that the quality of competitors' services is not good. Survival—personal and organizational—at any cost becomes the watchword.

These behaviors are not only unethical; they are suicidal. If we have learned nothing else from the recent flood of analyses of orga-nizational effectiveness, we should understand that acting on the basis of sound moral principles is key to success.

I do not think it is a coincidence that Johnson & Johnson, which manufactures Tylenol, is both very successful and has an ongoing organizational commitment to honesty and ethical behav-ior. This was evident in their extraordinary response to the Tylenol poisonings in Chicago. Johnson & Johnson did not try to protect its competitive edge by demanding that the product stay on the shelves, thus risking further tragedy. The firm wanted the public protected first, and took an enormous financial risk in withdrawing Tylenol from the market. When the drug was reintroduced in tamper-proof containers, it regained its earlier popularity. And Johnson & Johnson was seen as courageous and socially conscious.

It seems to me that morality in leadership is not only desirable, it is essential—especially in competitive or adversarial environments. Viscount Nelson knew that. He understood that organizational survival can be achieved through courage, commitment, vision and by staying close to one's conscience. Nelson was killed at Trafalgar, but his fleet and his country were victorious, which was his ultimate goal.

Nelson not only triumphed, he became a hero for all time. One reason for this was his ability to see beyond the selfish concerns of the moment to the larger cause and the longer view. He teaches us that in the end, we will be judged by the consequences of our decisions. Pursuing the momentary ethics of convenience will not serve today's leaders well when that judgment comes. As Winston Churchill once said, "The only guide to a man is his conscience; the only shields to his memory are the rectitude and sincerity of his actions."

Doing the Wrong Thing

Failure in Ethics

September 1988

Can there be failure in ethical decision-making? As more healthcare organizations accept ethics not only as a component of pastoral care and patient counseling, but as a matter of good management, this is worth asking. In other words, can you do the wrong thing in the course of doing the right thing?

Now, many people—including me—would argue that it is unfair to measure ethical success or failure with the same yardstick used for other management activities. It is difficult to think of lumping the ethics committee or ethics education in with, say, productivity measures or risk management. Ethics is, after all, a qualitative field, not a quantitative one.

Furthermore, ethical decision-making includes many people who are not formally trained in ethics, such as caregivers, patients and their families, trustees, and members of administrative staffs. Relatively few of these people are driven by mad *professional* ambition to succeed in their ethics considerations; they see this activity as voluntary and personal. Still, I think they want to do well in their pursuit of ethics.

How can success and failure in healthcare ethics be defined? There are two tiers of ethics activities—*organizational* and *individual*. In organizational ethics activities, several types of failure can be identified:

- **Failure to accept ethics as a legitimate concern.**
  Inertia, conservatism, or fear on the part of the
  organization (or of individuals) can lead to denial
  of the validity of ethics as an organizational concern.
  But risk-taking, both personal and professional, is a
  necessary part of ethics.

- **Failure to learn.** If education, discussion, and consultations are all taking place, but the same problems
  remain and/or recur, then the ethics effort may be serving only as a form of organizational window dressing.

- **Failure to develop process.** Ethics activities should not
  be based on seat-of-the-pants, crisis-oriented actions
  on the part of a few individuals. Although an ethics
  effort is almost always initiated by a small number of
  people—often only one or two—those individuals do
  not an ethics program make. A committed organization
  develops process, so that the ethics effort will survive
  even if its initiators depart.

- **Failure to be realistic.** The mere presence of an ethics
  committee, ethics consultant, or ethics training will
  not solve all the ethical problems everyone is having.
  Ethics activities offer a means of solving problems; they
  are not an end in themselves.

On an *individual* level, these failures can occur, but there are
other pitfalls:

- **Failure to think broadly.** Most ethical dilemmas
  involve conflicts of values. Thus, a successful resolution
  does not mean forcing your values on others, but rather
  reaching a consensus that leaves all parties comfortable
  with the result.

- **Failure to consider context.** Much of the ethics literature focuses on individual cases and "micro" situations. But no individual goes through life without a context—social, historical, and cultural. Decisions should be made with some consciousness of society's interest and the general welfare—present and future.

- **Failure to accept frustration.** H. Tristram Engelhardt, MD, PhD, of Baylor University, points out that there is a difference between what is unfortunate and what is unfair. There are unfortunate events about which we can do nothing, he says; but there are also unfair events that can be prevented. Ethical energy should focus on what can be changed.

In ethics as in clinical care, sometimes even when the operation is a success, the patient dies. If we have tried mightily, and have done our best to achieve a good and ethical result, we have not failed; the only failure is if we lose faith, blame ourselves, or stop trying.

• • • • • • •

This article originally contained a poem for which we were unable to obtain reprint permission.

Marketing and Fear

January 1989

I encountered an interesting question of marketing morality last year while I was speaking on ethics and healthcare quality at a meeting. I showed a videotape of a television spot produced by Mount Sinai Hospital Medical Center in Chicago. It depicts a pregnant woman in a rowboat who is, literally, up a creek without a paddle. As she tries to propel the boat with her bare hands in the rapid current, the narrator says that women who have been told they must undergo cesarean section should know that they will have options as to how their babies can be delivered. Interested women are invited to call a number at Mount Sinai for further information.

I think it's a great spot; but a woman in the audience criticized it. She said it seeks to frighten potential patients, and that her organization would never use that approach. I responded that I thought there was a distinction between the use of fear to provide information about important options (as the Mount Sinai tape did), and using fear to sell products or services that might be marginal.

Since then, I've been thinking about that exchange. And I would like to share a couple of thoughts about the specific issue of scaring patients as a means of marketing a product or service.

In the first place, we must acknowledge that a great deal of American marketing is based on fear: fear of unwanted body hair, bad breath, having your home disparaged by the neighbors, or having your wallet or car stolen, to name a few. I think that's why many

Americans do not consider advertising and marketing as the most forthright activities in our economy.

Yet the public does accept the use of fear in one form of health-care marketing: public health messages. Education campaigns about the risks of smoking, the spread of acquired immune deficiency syndrome (AIDS), and seat belt use are familiar to all of us; and all of them use fear as a persuasive device. Sometimes, as in efforts to promote better dental hygiene, what started out as a public health campaign has now become part and parcel of commercial advertising.

Why do we accept scare tactics in public health messages when we question them in other advertising? I think it is because we believe, deep down, that public health authorities have our best interests at heart. They are unlikely to be motivated by the promise of profit; in fact, in seeking better health behaviors, they are actually trying to *decrease* their business. They don't seem to want our money (not directly, anyway). So we assume that there is an altruistic basis to their scare tactics.

This belief in the ethical basis of public health campaigns continues, despite the fact that these ads can and do produce unintended adverse effects. The campaign against smoking has produced millions of individuals whose attitude toward smokers is not one of peers desiring to protect the smoker, but rather of paternalistic superiors desiring to oppress the smoker. This often reinforces the rebellion that underlies some people's tenacious insistence on continuing the habit. (It also ignores the conclusion of the head of the Public Health Service, C. Everett Koop, MD, that smoking is an addiction.)

Public health campaigns against AIDS, needless to say, have inadvertently helped fuel the hysteria surrounding that disease. And seat belt campaigns have led to a libertarian protest against required use; this sparked a referendum that repealed compulsory seat belt use in Massachusetts, a state usually characterized by strong public health regulation.

Nevertheless, it seems that Americans will accept healthcare marketing that is frightening when they believe that the marketers are trying to protect them. Thus the ethics lessons for healthcare marketers in the private sector are clear:

- Do not use fear in order to sell a product or service so much as to encourage sensible, self-protective health behavior.

- *Never* be dishonest, or even come close to being dishonest, in marketing healthcare; it will come back to haunt you in this consumerist age.

- Evaluate every proposed marketing campaign in light of the question, "For whose good do we seek this result? Ours or that of those we hope to serve?" (We all like to think that those two interests are consonant, but this is not always the case.)

- If you are marketing an optional, marginal, or cosmetic service, do not attempt to promote it in the same way in which necessary core services are marketed. Consumers are not stupid, and "scare-tactic" marketing of liposuction (such as suggesting that a woman's husband will leave her if she does not undergo "body sculpting") will backfire. In fact, such an approach could wreck campaigns for periodic mammography exams and similar services that can be vital to good health.

Remember that the public bias is *against*, not for, the marketer; therefore, the best way to *appear* ethical in marketing is to *be* ethical in marketing.

Copycats, Copycats

July 1989

Maybe it's because I don't understand a lot of technology. Maybe it has to do with the fact that some religions prohibit capturing a person's image on film, tape, or even in a mirror. Or maybe it's traceable to my concern that we are becoming passive spectators of our own lives, thanks to the pervasiveness of television and other noninteractive communications media.

Whatever the reason, I find myself growing more and more uncomfortable with how communications resources are used in healthcare. Specifically, I question the wanton use—without adequate safeguards or rules—of photocopying, audiotape, and videotape.

Much of my discomfort stems from ethical concerns. Now, these may not be world-shaking ethics issues; they are not as global as rationing nor as agonizing as termination of treatment. But they are ethics issues nonetheless, and are worthy of at least passing consideration.

So what's the problem? This is the electronics age! These tools make life a lot easier. I certainly concur. When I was in college, back in the Dark Ages, if I missed a class and asked to copy someone's notes, it literally meant that I would have to copy that person's notes by hand. And I can't complain about being able to tape a favorite movie that comes on at 2 a.m., rather than trying to force myself to stay up and watch it. But when it comes to healthcare education, patient care, and medical records, I think the stakes are higher.

Information Can Hurt

Too often, I am asked to participate in a private, informal discussion, only to find that a videotape camera or tape recorder has been erected to document the grand moment. The person seeking to make the recording always assures me that the recording is for "private use only," and won't be used for profit-making purposes.

That misses the point. Like everyone else, I have a right to privacy, and becoming part of someone else's "private" tape library, unless I have volunteered to do so, is a violation of my personal and professional privacy.

More important, pressuring patients to be videotaped, for educational or other purposes, treads on very shaky ethical ground. Most patients (or employees) are reluctant to turn down the people who are treating them or who employ them. Besides, being a hospital patient involves such a massive loss of privacy that being taped seems to be only one more minor indignity.

The problem is, that indignity may become public. I once watched videotaped interviews of several people who had undergone delicate reproductive surgery. These tapes were then shown, as an educational exercise, to people who worked in the same organization as the people who had been taped. Members of the audience were giggling at the people they knew. Although the patients had given their permission to be taped, I doubt they knew how much their privacy would be compromised.

Audiotaping and videotaping of patients or other people in a healthcare setting should be done only after frank discussion of the exact uses to which the tapes will be put. And great care must be taken to assure the potential subject that no prejudice will attach to his or her refusal to be taped.

Confidentiality

During a Chicago mayoral election a few years ago, news came out that one of the candidates had been treated for severe depression.

The information came from his medical records, which had been leaked to the press by a hospital employee. This was cited as a contributing factor to his losing the election.

Today, information that a patient, fellow worker, or medical staff member has tested positive for human immunodeficiency virus (HIV) can have devastating results for that person's employment status, ability to acquire or retain health insurance, and personal or professional relationships, should it fall into the wrong hands.

Someone who has died of an "embarrassing" disease may not have wanted that information splashed all over the papers. Yet too many hospitals have become sieves through which highly sensitive information sifts out to other employees, reporters, insurers, relatives, and attorneys. The photocopier has made this easy.

What also makes it easy is lack of organizational respect for the confidentiality of privileged information. It is difficult to stop gossip, but it is certainly possible to prevent it from getting started. That requires a top-level commitment.

Such a commitment has been made by Joseph Swedish, president of Mary Washington Hospital in Fredericksburg, Virginia. He passes out a card to new employees. It states the hospital's mission and standards of care, then closes with a short section on confidentiality: "Care enough to respect the power of information and its potentially harmful effect on each other, our patients, and their families. Information can hurt; treat it wisely!" That includes wise treatment of duplication of private material, whether potentially damaging or not.

Get It in Writing

The issue of permission involves legal as well as ethical considerations. If you want to take my picture, audiotape my words, or make a videotape or movie of me, *get my permission first*. And get it in writing.

Too often, someone who would automatically seek a signed release for still photography thinks nothing of setting up tape recorders or videotape cameras without getting the permission of those involved. That can lead to lawsuits; it is also extremely rude, and certainly violates basic ethical tenets. So does copying and distributing tapes made for private use, without the approval of the subject of the tape.

Overuse of duplicating technologies also encourages laziness in teaching and learning. It is easy for a teacher or physician or whomever to toss a tape onto a machine for the patient or student to watch; with television so prominent in our lives, we are used to this method of learning. But when it comes to patient decision-making, professional education, and other areas in which person-to-person contact is necessary, electronic teaching tools are at best ancillary to the main event, which is one person helping another.

Despite the development of very sophisticated, intelligent video aids in patient education and informed consent, I still believe that most patients, faced with a difficult decision, will watch the tape, then turn to the physician and ask, "So what do you think, Doc?" That these technologies are marvelous *aids* is indisputable; that they can replace the personal interactions that are the guts of healthcare is doubtful.

Finally, there are those people who use the office photocopier for personal work. Although this is theft, I believe that most of the miscreants do not really intend to steal. They do it for convenience; it's much less bother to use the office copier than to troop out in the snow or heat on one's lunch hour to use a commercial machine.

I suggest that a box be placed next to the machine, with a note asking that personal copying be done before or after work or during lunch and break time, and that a donation of 5 or 10 cents per page be left in the box. The money can be earmarked for indigent care or a healthcare charity. I think this is preferable to the time-consuming, frustrating, and ultimately useless exercise of trying to keep people from using the machine.

We are all becoming copycats, and I have no desire to see these exceptional technologies eliminated or restricted unduly. But we must be aware that these are only machines; they are as good or as bad as we allow them to be. They have no ethical values themselves; we folks must supply that element of this exciting, but ethically dangerous, technological revolution.

This Thing About Machines

September 1989

When I was a child, I was enthralled by Rod Serling's "Twilight Zone" television series. One episode in particular still sticks in my mind. Entitled "A Thing About Machines," it concerned a man who hated and abused his technological possessions. Eventually, his machines fought back; his electric razor chased him through the house, his kitchen appliances rebelled, and his car finally murdered him by drowning him in his own swimming pool.

I was struck by that episode because I am what might be called a technology incompetent. I don't understand how anything works; not electricity, computers, telephones, fiberoptics, or anything else along that line. I use them—they are indispensable—but my relationship with them is based on faith, not comprehension.

Perhaps for this reason, I have a lot of sympathy for patients who are confronted with technological healthcare. I understand why healthcare machinery clashes with their concept of care, which probably involves either nursing and kindness, or else surgery and white-robed doctor-priests. But few people, when you say "healthcare" to them, envision an MRI, linear accelerator, or CT scanner. They don't think of it in those terms because they don't want to think of it in those terms.

It's important to understand patients' fear of healthcare technology in order to formulate a humane response. Several factors are involved. First, it is rare that the application of a machine to a human body has a painless and positive result. Usually, when we see or read news about machines and people, the reports are of guns, knives, cattle prods, and the like. It is not coincidental that one of the most famous horror-gore films of all time was *The Texas Chainsaw Massacre*, which involved the misapplication of a technology to a gruesome end. We just don't think bodies and machines are very compatible.

Steel Contraptions

Second, virtually all of us have experienced at least one form of technological healthcare: dentistry. And we don't like it much. I cannot recall anyone telling me what a swell time he or she had at the dentist's office. Indeed, the success of dentists in promoting better dental health is due as much to a fear of the alternative as to a born-again desire to take care of one's teeth. That fear probably underlay the willingness of American communities to allow fluoridation of their drinking water—quite a threatening proposal at the time.

But we fear dentistry not only because it can hurt—after all, giving blood can hurt—but also because the pain is accompanied by what sounds like a chainsaw, as well as a variety of other steel contraptions that don't look friendly at all. Remember that Dustin Hoffman, in *Marathon Man,* was tortured with a dentist's drill.

Third, there is a frightening loss of control involved in being treated by machines. You may not like or trust your nurse or physician, but you hope that you can reason with him or her, ask questions, and exert some control. It's extremely difficult to ask a linear accelerator what it's doing, or why it is doing it, or what the effect of what it is doing will be. Furthermore, some healthcare technologies render the patient virtually incommunicado; as a friend of mine said of hyperbaric chambers, "You might as well be in a coffin." Serving as a bit of "throughput" for a scanner that resembles a sausage machine is not likely to enhance one's sense of security, either.

"It Could Be Worse"

Fourth, many patients feel violated when these machines invade their bodies—and sometimes, even when they don't. A disturbing essay by Margo Kaufman in the May 1, 1989 *Newsweek*, told of her experiences as a breast cancer patient. She tells of being prepared for radiation therapy: "I winced as the radiation therapist drew what looked like a flow chart across my chest and ordered me not to remove it until the end of treatment. 'You don't look very happy,' the technician marveled. Happy? I felt as if I'd been raped by a felt-tip pen!. . .Yet nobody even seemed aware that this process was dehumanizing. 'It could be worse,' I was reminded. 'In some clinics, you get tattooed.'"

Patients undergo barium enemas, gastroscopy, laparoscopy, myriad forms of surgery, pelvic examinations, intubation. These are violations, and are perceived as such. Modern consumer preference for non-invasive treatments is as much a matter of self-protection as of belief in the efficacy of those treatments.

The fifth factor involves the issue of familiarity. Most people who work in healthcare know all about technology, and how it works, and what it does, and how useful it is. We become inured to the big machines, the whirs and clicks and buzzes, the felt-tip pens, the weird images in the dim light of the cathode ray tube. To a degree, we must become inured; healthcare is a profession, and to be a professional means acquiring what physicians term "detached concern." But to be detached does not mean being callous. Margo Kaufman tells us in her essay: "The instant some pathologist, whom you've never met, looks through a microscope and delivers a verdict that your tumor is malignant, your life is in the hands of medical professionals, whom in most cases you don't know but you're still supposed to trust."

"True, when you get on an airplane, you're making a similar leap of faith. You're putting your life in the hands of a pilot whom you've never seen, who is flying a plane that for all you know may have a defective door latch. *But at least the airlines recognize that you might be worried. Their entire staff minimizes your fears. They may not reassure you, but at least they recognize the problem and make an effort."* [Italics mine.] She does not find the same true of the treatment of cancer patients by the healthcare system.

Adjusting the Mindset

So what is the ethical, professional way to deal with patient fear of technology? Much of the answer lies in the mindset of the caregiver, a mindset that needs adjusting. To wit:

Just because a patient's fears are irrational doesn't mean they should not be addressed. For example, I am terrified of airline turbulence. I know it's harmless; I know if my seat belt is buckled, I will not be hurt; I know it's part of flying. It still scares me. If each of us can recognize an irrational fear of our own (turbulence, snakes, spiders, thunderstorms, whatever), it will help us understand patients who fear machines that go bump in the night, even if they know those machines are helpful. Many hospitals have programs designed to allay the fears of pediatric patients, yet do little to allay the fears of adult patients, because we presume they know all about what is going to happen to them. They don't.

A little explanation never hurts. Patients, especially those who are used to paternalistic healthcare, may not ask about the technology that is used on them. That does not mean they do not wish to know about it. They may be afraid to ask, or to be thought fools for asking. Informed consent must include a reasonable explanation of what the technology is, how it works, what it does, and why it is being used. It is not enough to tell the patient that "we need to run this test." Patients deserve more information than that.

Don't lie in order to calm an agitated patient. It is not ethically defensible to lie to a patient, or to withhold information, because you think the patient will freak out if told the truth. Take the traditional description of giving blood: fast, easy, and painless. It is none of the three. It takes about an hour, plus travel time; it is easy only if the technician is competent, which is not always the case; and it is not painless, although the dull ache and needle-stick are minor. But we should not lie about it. Similarly, mammograms are uncomfortable; many radiological procedures are worse; some tests hurt. I think patients feel less betrayed if they know what they are in for than if they are told it will be a picnic, and it turns out to be the Texas Barium Massacre.

Technology should never be used spuriously. Current cost containment efforts focus on "big-ticket" surgical procedures like organ transplants. The guns are also pointed at laboratory tests, although the argument appears to concern profiteering more than appropriateness. Between those two poles is a world of "little-ticket" technology, both therapeutic and diagnostic. But these "middle" technologies are no less vulnerable to inappropriate use than are their higher-profile cousins.

An Ethical Mandate

We must keep reminding ourselves: Healthcare is not always benign or harmless. It can be painful, frightening, dangerous, even crippling or fatal, not to mention expensive. As new technologies offer both higher risks and better outcomes, it becomes even more ethically imperative that we learn, not just how to use them, but also when and why to use them. Otherwise we are subjecting patients to needless fear and risk for economic or ego reasons. That is about as violent a violation of the ethics of healthcare as one can commit.

Does this mean that we should become what George Will described as "health care Luddites," recalling the hand weavers who, faced with automated looms, smashed them? Hardly. But we must understand that the increasingly technological basis of healthcare is accompanied by an ethical mandate.

Rather than distancing us from patients and enhancing professional detachment, new and old technologies alike require us to form even closer relationships with patients, to make a greater commitment to understanding and allaying their fears, and to have a firmer determination to use technology only when its use is indicated. To do otherwise dehumanizes not only patients, but also the caregivers in whom they have placed their trust.

Loose Ends

November 1989

There are those among us who don't notice even their own birthdays; I, on the other hand, take note of many anniversaries, whether they are mine, or somebody else's, or society's. I am also one of those people who just can't let a decade go without clutching at it, trying to suck its juices and digest it down to an understandable morsel. So, as we close in on the end of that troublesome time known as the Eighties, I feel compelled to comment on its probable legacy.

This last year of the decade—1989—has marked a large number of significant anniversaries. On September 1, 1939, the Nazis invaded Poland and thus forced the beginning of World War II. That same year, the town of Cooperstown, New York, talked major league baseball into setting up the Hall of Fame in that hamlet. The US Congress was born 100 years ago, the French republic 200 years ago. Other celebrations this year have included the twentieth birthday of "Monday Night Football" and of the Woodstock rock festival, the seventy-fifth birthday of Wrigley Field in Chicago, and the fiftieth birthday of the film version of *Gone with the Wind*. Each of these occasions has been scrutinized, with greater or lesser solemnity, by analysts and scholars seeking to determine What It All Meant.

Of Baseball, Ships, and Healthcare Ethics

I see 1989 marking two other milestones, both producing lessons that are directly applicable to the pursuit and practice of ethics in healthcare: (1) In August 1989, one of the greatest baseball players who ever lived, Pete Rose, accepted banishment from the game as punishment for having gambled on sports and allegedly on baseball and even his own team, and (2) on April 28, 1989, we marked the bicentennial anniversary of the mutiny on the *Bounty*. What do these events teach us about healthcare ethics?

Rose's supporters complained, pointing out that Babe Ruth was a womanizer and a boozer, that Ty Cobb seemed to take pleasure in injuring opposing players, and that other ball players have philandered, gambled, and cheated. These complaints did not take into account what major league baseball did take into account: The rules have changed.

In 1919, when several Chicago White Sox players threw the World Series, they paid for it. In more recent decades, the public (and baseball) looked the other way as sports heroes behaved in less than heroic ways. But now the rules have changed again, and morality is back in style. As a result, Pete Rose will pay a heavy price for what many others had gotten away with.

Similarly, the rules have changed for healthcare ethics. This is no longer untried ground, where every decision is new, every incident is ground-breaking, every effort is innovative. We have gained a body of experience, of law, of public opinion, that we can use as a guide.

This means that now, in many situations—death and dying, informed consent, clinical research—we can spend as much time educating, informing, and spreading the word as we have spent agonizing as we tiptoed over virgin ground. We have some new rules now; we should learn them.

And the mutiny on the *Bounty*? I have thought much about what it can teach us. Contrary to those who see in the story grand schemes of life and death, authority and rebellion, freedom and slavery, I see a landscape of choices.

A group of sailors and officers had to decide whether to break the most solemn oath of all: the promise to obey orders. Each man had to decide with whom to cast his lot—the captain, Bligh, or the rebel, Christian. Those who stayed with Bligh were forced into open boats and sailed over thousands of miles of unforgiving ocean to safety. Those who sided with Christian had to decide whether to debark in Tahiti or to sail on to parts unknown. Those who chose Tahiti were caught and eventually hanged. Those who chose Christian and Pitcairn's Island lived out the rest of their lives in a place so mismarked on the charts that they knew they would never see home again.

Their epic tale is not unlike our more mundane lives, for the moral is the same: Life is full of difficult choices with very high stakes. And despite all that has occurred in healthcare, I still think that trying to do the right thing, the path that seems morally right, is the best policy, no matter what the consequences. That principle becomes harder to follow as the choices become more murky and the consequences more grave, but its attraction remains undiminished.

Milestones in a Singular Era

In healthcare ethics, the decade of the Eighties has been a singular era. We witnessed the deaths of Karen Ann Quinlan and countless other individuals whose lives were no longer meaningful for them or the people who loved them—and whose passing bred new rights and new responsibilities for others. We saw the continuing passionate debate over the rights of fetuses, disabled newborns, and mothers, more fervent now than ever.

We gained the report of the President's Commission for the Study of Ethical Problems in Medicine and Biomedical and Behavioral Research, which produced a "first cut" at a daunting array of issues and was one of the first efforts to include access to care as an ethics problem. Everyone involved deserves hosannas, but Alexander Morgan Capron, the commission's executive director (now a professor at the University of Southern California), deserves special praise for having stuck with it, rather than chucking it all in favor of a Buddhist monastery somewhere along the way.

There were many other milestones, from the introduction of rationing of care into the language of everyday ethics to the Rudy Linares case, in which a distraught young father disconnected his comatose infant son from hospital life support and gained, unexpectedly, the forgiveness and even the backing of a large part of the nation (not to mention a cheerleading press). The times have indeed changed from a decade before.

As the decade dwindles to a close, it seems that mountains have been moved, but the process has been subtle. It is as though we looked up one day and found that the skyline had been permanently altered. These are the major alterations:

- Paternalism toward patients on the part of providers is only acceptable now when patients select that form of relationship, as a voluntary choice.

- Social concerns—confidentiality, access to care, justice in the allocation of resources—are as much a part of ethics as are the concerns of the individual patient.

- Competent patients almost always have the right to dictate the circumstances of their care, whether providers agree with their choices or not.

- The use of healthcare technology is no longer an automatic good, and is subject to the scrutiny and choices of patients.

- Like it or not, the courts are part of ethics decision-making; the extent of their role will depend on how much power patients and providers are willing to concede to them.

Because of these and other changes, future ethics decisions and issues will be tougher than they were in the past. Expedient answers will be proposed and in some cases implemented, but this will prove disastrous, and more thoughtful problem-solving will prevail. This situation reminds me of the words of William Campbell, MD, a St.

Louis physician, who observed that "most of the cheap and easy diseases have been taken care of."

There were some relatively easy issues in the earlier days of ethics, like the fact that competent patients should not be forced to undergo care they do not want and from which they cannot benefit. Issues in the future are going to be a lot less cut and dried.

An Ethic for the Nineties

What has been gained? We may not know that for a while. What we have learned will not remain as a collection of random facts and cases and incidents. The bits of information will eventually fuse into an amalgam or a synthesis that is far more useful. I do believe that during the Nineties we will benefit from what we have learned and synthesized during this turbulent, sometimes frightful, often unkind decade. At the moment we are digesting, amalgamating, and making sense of it all, and what we come up with will be the basis of the healthcare ethic of the Nineties.

What we can see now are the outlines of that ethic. We must forge a new relationship between provider (institutional or individual) and patient, with a pronounced power shift toward the patient. We need to extend the ethics of justice and caring beyond those we gladly treat to those whom we treat grudgingly or not at all, so that we can come to a balance between our attitude toward the cash-paying liposuction patient and our attitude toward the uninsured, indigent AIDS patient who begs at the door.

We are going to have to create a new ethic to address what genetics research, transplant technology, molecular biology, and other wonders are asking us. Yet we must maintain a continuum—a holding of hands across time—with those who struggled with ethics questions in the past, so that our new rules build upon the foundation our predecessors created out of their own personal and professional agonies.

Let us make the Nineties a time of moving forward in healthcare ethics, a time in which we can take pride. And let us do that by acknowledging what we did wrong, and right, during the Eighties.

Marginal Missions
and Missionary Margins

January 1990

It became one of the stock hospital phrases of the 1980s, having first been used (so legend has it) by the sisters who govern Catholic hospitals: "no margin, no mission." If the hospital cannot cover its costs and get a little bit ahead in order to have reserves, it cannot remain open, and its ability to fulfill its mission will, of necessity, be destroyed.

But the phrase moved beyond concerned religious orders to become a commonly used, and soon overused, capsule defense of hospital economic behavior. Today it is a glib—indeed, smug—rebuke to anyone who suggests that hospitals might not be doing all they can to husband the resources society has granted them.

It seems to me that a closer examination of the mission-margin relationship is in order, for three reasons. First, when the inspector general of the Department of Health and Human Services, assorted congressmen and senators, consumer advocates, and, increasingly, the press continue to suggest that hospitals are profiteering on Medicare and other programs, it behooves hospitals to respond with something more persuasive than dubious margin statistics and a perfunctory "no margin, no mission."

Second, the fact that some sort of margin is necessary, which few people would dispute, does not mean that any margin, no matter how inflated or how cruelly achieved, is automatically necessary and morally justified. Doing well is not necessarily the same as doing good. There is quite a spectrum between the need for a hospital to balance its books and the Machiavellian pursuit of the highest possible margin. Margin and mission are related, but to claim that the margin is the mission is to pervert the notion of mission.

Third, providers can no longer claim the high moral ground simply by virtue of being providers. This is a dearly held self-deception throughout healthcare; I am a doctor (or nurse, or hospital administrator, or HMO executive, or clinic director), and therefore anything I do is morally good, because I am doing it. This delusion has allowed physicians to commit butchery, hospitals to engage in sociopathic behavior, and nurses to violate the rights of patients, without guilt. Similarly, hospitals like to think that anything they do in pursuit of their missions is automatically good, because their missions (which are defined in eloquent and high-minded language on a plaque in the lobby) are good. Whether its mission is relevant or appropriate to the community the hospital serves, and whether the mission is honored in a more than casual manner (if at all) is not important. It is the form, not the substance, that counts.

With American hospitals at a crossroads in terms of their future (including, in the eyes of some pessimists, the issue of whether they *have* a future), it is not sufficient to say, "I gotta have a margin because I must fulfill my wonderful mission, so give me more money and leave me alone." They will neither give you more money nor leave you alone. And it is entirely possible that they should not do either, because you may not deserve it.

Trappings of Charity

This change in public attitudes has been difficult for hospitals, because they have long worn the trappings of charity—the mission to serve the sick and the poor, the white cloak of voluntarism, the high principles of social service, the ivoried morality of science. And, to be fair, it is not entirely hospitals' fault that they still see themselves in this light. This was the light in which society saw them for a long time.

In her brilliant portrait of the American hospital in the 20th century (*In Sickness and in Wealth*, Basic Books, 1989), Professor Rosemary Stevens points out that hospitals today are still often seen as what they were at the beginning of the century: "institutions through which the moral values of American society are expressed." Americans still have great hope for the moral purity of their hospitals—on the social level, because these are great social institutions with a proud heritage, and on the individual level, because we are all potential patients, and we want to feel safe within their walls.

But if hell hath no fury like a woman scorned, a society scorned is a close runner-up. And society is beginning to think that the moral purity of hospitals ain't what it used to be (it probably never was what society thought it was, but that's another story). To a degree, this is a bum rap; as Professor Stevens also notes, it is unfair to encourage hospitals to behave like businesses, imbued with market mania and primed for cutthroat competition, and then to condemn them when they succeed in doing so. Nevertheless, hospitals were eager to undertake the role of hard-edged business enterprise, and very easily slid into the use of industrial terminology, marketing campaigns, and disdain for and avoidance of the poor, insured and uninsured alike.

The Tax Man

No sane observer could have truly believed that this embracing of mercenary attitudes would go unchallenged, and it has not. The tax man has responded with a simple and logical equation: Act like a business, pay taxes like a business. It is really quite sad that it has taken the Internal Revenue Service, certainly one of the most hated institutions in the country, to remind what were once some of the most beloved institutions in the country of what they are supposed to be about.

Government has played another key role in the confusion over margin and mission. In undertaking the subsidy of hospital care of virtually all the elderly and between one-third and one-half of those living in poverty, government seemed to obviate the need for broad charitable behavior on the part of hospitals.

In sparking this "death of charity," as Professor Stevens dubs it, government greatly lessened what had been seen as the primary charitable mission of hospitals: care of the poor and vulnerable. Then what were they supposed to do? It reminds me of the question asked by Henry James after Karl Marx alleged that God was dead: "What is the role of faith if there is no God to have faith in?"

Confused about which god to follow, hospitals fell in with bad company and embraced Mammon. Too often, mission became marginal, a set of knee-jerk phrases that could not be fulfilled—a discrepancy that went unnoticed because no one was trying to fulfill them. Likewise, in the absence of a mission to guide its use, the margin began to be spent in inappropriate ways. Far from being used in a missionary manner, margins were frittered away on risky new ventures, servicing of unnecessary debt, and bloated administrative overhead.

All this was a warning; but we do not always heed warnings. The development of the atomic bomb was code-named "Trinity." Years later, asked when talks on nuclear arms control should have begun, J. Robert Oppenheimer, the physicist who ran the project, said, "The day after Trinity." Similarly, discussion of the relationship of margin and mission should have begun 25 years ago, as Medicare appeared on the horizon and promised to change hospital financing forever.

Start the Discussion

Well, better late than never; let's start the discussion now, in every organization, *beginning on the board level*. Ownership is not an issue; public, voluntary, and proprietary organizations alike need to engage in this kind of introspection. Whether an organization pays taxes or not is an issue of tax status, not a measure of its commitment to mission or its right to a margin. I suggest the following thoughts to help frame the discussion.

Does the organization know what its losses and margin really are? I recently completed a study of hospital uncompensated care for the *Journal of the American Medical Association,* and my greatest frustration was the constant use of inflated figures for uncompensated care, based on billed charges (which virtually no one pays) and listed as "deductions from revenue." Hospitals also report two margins, one for patient care revenue and one for non-patient care revenue. This statistical sleight of hand is self-serving and vaguely dishonest; it is also unpersuasive evidence in the court of public opinion. Every organization should know how much it is making and losing, and should share that information openly and in an understandable way.

Margins involve both revenue and expense. One of the manifest ironies of the 1980s is that healthcare expenditures have increased more than 100 percent in this decade, and no one can really explain why. Even someone as notoriously pro-hospital as I cannot defend that rate of increase, especially when I see the massive architectural projects, the boutique services, the vice-presidential limousines, the lavish expense accounts, the advertising budgets, the estimated $25 billion going into the passive hands of stockholders, and the duplication, everywhere the duplication of services and technology. If an organization needs to increase its margin, it should ask itself whether the first sacrifice should be care of uninsured pregnant women—or the retreat and golf outing at the Ritz-Carlton.

Doing as little as possible is not mission fulfillment. Somewhere along the line, hospitals convinced themselves that if they fulfilled their Hill-Burton obligations, they were fully honoring their mission of serving the poor and downtrodden. However, charity and mission fulfillment are not simply what you can get away with. Minimum requirements are just that: minimal. They are floors, and should not become ceilings.

A social service mission extends beyond the self-interest of the organization. I once knew a cynic who explained the conservatism of foundations by saying, "The purpose of any foundation is to protect the assets of the foundation." Similarly, most hospitals believe the single most important issue in the mission-versus-margin debate is the survival of the organization: "We can't help anybody if we're closed." This assumes that every institution's survival represents an ethical good.

I would be the first to claim, with passion, that some needed hospitals have closed; I *know* that some needed hospitals have closed. But I would also be the first to claim that quite a few unnecessary hospitals are still around.

Despite institutional pride, tradition, the hospital-as-employer argument, and, often, community support, some hospitals could probably best fulfill their missions by closing and freeing up resources for other health and social services. To state unequivocally that the first loyalty of a healthcare organization must always be to itself is to state a highly questionable mission. It reminds me of the famous Vietnam War comment: "It was necessary to destroy the village in order to liberate it." If a healthcare organization purchases its survival at the price of its own honor or the community's health, then one must ask whom it thinks it is serving.

Any organization's mission is inextricably tied to the missions of its brethren. I find it amazing that at this point in the development of hospital consortia, alliances, and systems, the members of these organizations turn pale and gasp at the idea that the stronger ones should perhaps share resources with the weaker ones. I find it amazing that wealthy hospitals in affluent areas resist the notion that they owe something to the poor and the hospitals that serve them. Having fat reserves and big margins in upscale suburbs is not necessarily evidence of superb management; it may be evidence of market area. It should be apparent by now that either hospitals are going to voluntarily support each other (and yes, that includes the public hospitals), or government will force cross-subsidization.

Does the organization see itself as a vendor or as a charity? Professor Stevens argues that most hospitals play both roles. However, to claim to be a charity and to act only as a vendor is unacceptable. The organization has to know what it is, what it wants to be, and what its community wants it to be. Even if it cannot immediately fulfill all of its own and the community's expectations, the organization can at least give itself a star to shoot for.

Is the organization being honest about what it is and what it wants to do? I know of institutions with the usual pretty mission prose hanging on the wall whose CEOs say their real mission is to provide good care to the middle and upper classes. Period. I know of hospitals with little interest in serving the medically indigent; however, they pretend to care because they don't want it known that they do not care.

If you want to be strictly a business, without charitable pretension or intent, say so—and take the consequences. If you're afraid to do that, perhaps you should re-examine what you have chosen as goals. If you can't be proud of them, maybe you shouldn't be pursuing them. Mission cannot be a hidden agenda.

Are the uses to which the margin is put appropriate? The crux of the matter, of course, is the assumption that the margin that is obtained through effort, sacrifice, and brilliant management is carefully husbanded and used with innovation, conscience, and care. Is it? Too often, much of it is misspent. Or the margin is socked away, along with millions of dollars from previous years' margins, saved for a rainy day that somehow never comes, even as the infant mortality rate rises, the low-income elderly suffer, and epidemics eat their way through the poor. There never seems to be a need worthy of risking the accumulated funds.

It is precisely that attitude that got us into this mess. Too many hospitals made an inordinate amount of money, especially on Medicare, and then used it in questionable ways while access to care declined. Payers, unimpressed with how providers used their largesse, cut back to the point that many hospitals now are truly suffering. But as we blame the payers for their penury, let us remember that we squandered much of what we had, and now seem hypocritical in complaining that we are broke.

Delicate Equilibrium

The equilibrium between mission and margin will always be delicate. Some hospitals that have husbanded resources splendidly and served their communities generously and wisely will close. Some organizations that have been completely irrelevant since the day they started will prosper. Nevertheless, the best chance hospitals have to retain and/or reclaim the margins they need will be through meaningful, realistic missions that guide operations and budgeting. As Donald Berwick, MD, has said: "no mission, no margin."

The poet Louis MacNeice once wrote a magnificent love poem, "Flowers in the Interval." I would like to borrow that thought. For all those hospitals that have been missionary in the use of their margins and resistant to the marginal mission: flowers to you all, until justice comes to healthcare. For those who think that margin is more important than mission, or that margin is mission: May you understand that you are not only failing yourselves; your failure may drag all that is good in healthcare down with you.

The Perils of Detachment

March 1990

At one point in Bernard Pomerance's magnificent play, *The Elephant Man*, the terribly deformed hero, John Merrick, is having a discussion with his physician, Frederick Treves. Merrick is confused by Treves's harsh treatment of him after he sought to see a naked woman, an experience he had never had because women shunned him.

Treves tries to deflect his anger and begins talking about a woman patient upon whom he had once operated. Merrick asks him if he saw her naked. Treves replies, "When I was operating? Of course."

Merrick then asks, "Is it all right to see them naked if you cut them up afterwards?"

Treves replies, "I am a surgeon. It's just science; that's all it is. It's not love." Pressed further by Merrick, he finally says, "Love has got nothing to do with surgery. What difference does it make if I, or any other surgeon, loves a patient or not?"

Presence of a Victim

I was reminded of that exchange when I attended an unusual conference at Boston University a few weeks ago. It was entitled, "The Nazi Doctors and the Nuremberg Code: Relevance for Modern Medical Research." It was quite a gathering, and I could write reams about the thoughts it inspired. Perhaps someday I will.

For now, I want to concentrate on one of the many issues that were raised at the conference. It was expressed in two forms. The first was the eloquent, powerful presence of Eva Mozes Kor, who, along with her sister, was among the very few survivors of Joseph Mengele's horrific experiments on twins at Auschwitz-Birkenau. Both were injected with God-knows-what and observed, as experimenters waited for them to die. Eva recalls that, although she was only nine years old, she was determined not to give Mengele the satisfaction of watching her die. Perhaps that determination saved her.

Eva Kor sat at the conference and listened as a variety of speakers wrestled with the crimes of the Nazi physicians. Her presence gave life to the conceptual and theoretical models that were being defined and discussed. I think she made some speakers uncomfortable; it is easier, I suspect, to theorize about the academic ethical implications of genocidal crime and monstrous torture when one of the victims of those atrocities is not staring at you.

Eva Kor humanized the history and gave a personality and a voice to the grainy black-and-white films of the victims in the camps. She knows the enormous difference that can exist between love and surgery.

The second expression of the question occurred when Elie Wiesel, the Nobel laureate writer, poet, playwright, historian, and witness to the Holocaust, spoke for a few quiet moments. He stated that "the greatest shock of my life" was when he found, as he began his studies of the Holocaust, that so many physicians and intellectuals were involved in the conscious, willing perpetration of atrocities. These were the cream of Europe—educated at the best universities, trained in the finest hospitals. Yet 38,000 physicians (half the doctors in Germany) joined the Nazi party, and physicians were seven times as likely to join the SS as were members of the general population. "These were men who had studied for years," he said. "How could their education not shield them from evil?"

He answered his own question: These physicians hardened themselves against the humanity of their "patients." They were able to turn them into abstractions. "And when you turn human beings into abstractions," he warned, "they become meaningless."

The Thin Line

One slide shown at the conference will haunt me until I die. It is of a wartime research laboratory. One physician, in his SS uniform, busies himself with notes. A second physician, also in uniform, smiling, comforting, strokes a "patient"—as the man floats, helpless, suffering, in a tub of ice water while they freeze him to death. The physician probably satisfied himself that he was fulfilling his duty to his patient by comforting him as he killed him. As Wiesel also pointed out, most of these physicians did not believe they were doing wrong.

The idea that kept running through my mind was the traditional medical concept of "detached concern"—that thin line that physicians, nurses, orderlies, aides, and, for that matter, administrators and trustees, must tread between being too involved with patients, and too distant from them. It is a basic conflict of the caregiver: How can I be compassionate without becoming so involved that I cannot bear the suffering?

Nurses in burn units, physicians who care for AIDS patients, and social workers in transplant programs do burn out. Unable to find the balance between caring too much and caring too little, they come to care too much and eventually must absent themselves from the suffering in which they have become too involved.

The Nazi doctors went the other way. Having accepted insane concepts like "racial hygiene," the non-humanity of Jews and other ethnic groups, and the virtue of "pure science," they convinced themselves that totally dehumanizing patients simply made research easier. They argued, at their trials in Nuremberg, that the prisoners in the camps were doomed anyway, that all mankind would benefit from the results of their tortures, and, perhaps most horribly, that "scientists are not responsible for value judgments," a fallacy pointed out by Arthur Caplan, PhD, of the University of Minnesota, at the conference.

This last is a perverse expression of the quest for better patient care: What we find out, or the benefits that some other patient may reap, justify our torturing and murdering those in our care. No one need have worried that these physicians would become too involved in the suffering of their patients; they were causing it.

"A Universe in Every Person"

Asking how this could have happened, how men and women of medicine could debase themselves so thoroughly, Wiesel asserted that not only medical morality was called into question by the crimes of the Nazi doctors. So were "scholarship, learning, erudition, and culture," all of which must be re-examined in light of the massive failure of these scholarly, learned, erudite, and cultured men and women to honor basic concepts of decency.

To protect against such moral hardening in the future, he said, "We cannot see any person as an abstraction; we must see a universe in every person."

It is not always possible to see a universe in every person, especially every patient, when so many other factors intervene—the sheer number of patients, the short hospital stays that prevent bonding, one's own fatigue, cultural and other gaps between caregiver and patient, bad weather, irritating patient behaviors, and whether one's shoes fit. Often, love and surgery, indeed, have little or nothing to do with one another. But we must always keep in mind what can happen when patients become too dehumanized in the eye of the caregiver.

We must be utterly conscious of the dangers of not loving patients at all. We must guard against the creeping callousness that makes it easier for us to provide bad care, or no care at all. When patients cease to be people, everything is lost. That is how the cream of European medicine came to see torture as science. No matter the personal, professional, or financial cost, we must never allow ourselves to become that hard again.

. . . .

Millennium

Old Troubles for New

May 1990

Someone once defined marriage as a way of exchanging a bunch of old, tired problems for just as many new, exciting problems. Similarly, a surgeon once described organ transplantation, with all the immune system problems and medications that come with it, as replacing an acute disease with a chronic one.

Indeed, when most change occurs, we are less likely to get rid of our problems than we are to replace them with others.

This is especially true of bioethics, which, as the healthcare system undergoes massive change, promises as many dilemmas for the reconfigured system as for the old one. In fact, some of them will be worse. For although bioethics is a new field (at least in its expansion past the professional ethics of providers to questions involving patients and society), it is old enough to have a track record. That experience shows that ethics has concentrated on *relatively* easy issues—with great success, I might add.

To take one example: In a constitutional democracy such as ours, the fight over a patient's right to refuse treatment grew from a strong background of law, tradition, informal practice, and popular sentiment that pointed to one solution: the patient's right to choose.

This is not to say the struggle is over, or that it has been simple or fun—just that it has been easier than some other ethics debates that have not commanded so much attention. But the time is coming when most "easy" ethics issues will have been largely resolved, either by the courts or by custom and practice.

And as healthcare restructures itself (with a little help from its friends) into organizations rather than institutions, networks rather than buildings, and multiple levels and sites of care, a host of new ethics issues will appear. And some will be so perplexing as to remind us of Stephen Dunning's admonition, "Some haystacks don't even have any needle."

Here are a few of what may be the knotty ethics issues arising from the healthcare system that is now in the making:

Who Gets What When Everyone Has Coverage?

It seems obvious that within the next few years, the United States will extend access to care to all its citizens, probably by extending coverage. This will put many providers into the situation that public hospitals have faced for years: How should care be rationed when everyone is covered and the ability to pay cannot be used as a weeding-out device?

Many of our answers will come from county hospitals and military medicine. And the debate about "rationing of care"— which has largely been pursued by private-sector providers worried about relatively modest underpayments—is going to get real in a hurry.

How Should Genetic Information Be Used?

This area of research will breed some of the most horrifying questions of the twenty-first century, if not the 1990s.

The battle will likely proceed along two fronts. One will be access to and use of information concerning an individual's genetic predisposition to disease. We have at least one model: When a test for predisposition to Huntington's disease was developed, it was offered to members of families with a history of the disease, who had the right to refuse to take it.

However, with insurers trying to avoid covering anyone who might get sick, how long will it be before there is pressure to *force* people to undergo a battery of genetic tests to determine what they might get, and when?

Won't payers demand the information? Won't employers be interested in knowing if a worker is a candidate for early cancer? Even public health authorities might want the information in order to plan for future needs.

This will be a monstrous can of worms. And although we have the good model of the Huntington's approach, we also have the horrible model of the national hysteria over AIDS and the excesses it has bred in terms of violations of individual privacy.

The other battleground will be designer babies, which in turn will have two major components: prevention of problems and cosmetic improvements. If genetic testing shows that a fetus has a gene for some dread disease, should the pregnancy be terminated? Who decides what conditions would qualify? And do parents of modest means have the right to insist on having a disabled child whose care must be subsidized with public funds?

As for cosmetic changes, we can already stack the odds toward having a child of one sex or the other. Not far behind will be eye and hair color and adjustments in height and shoe size and heaven knows what else.

At the moment, one hospital that offers a program to increase the odds of having a male child does so only for those parents who are at disproportionate risk of having children with sex-linked genetic disease. I am not confident that such limits will last; there will be major attempts to market programs producing tall, slim, blond, blue-eyed, male children. Can lines be drawn? What will be the appropriate role for providers?

Who Is Responsible for the Patient?

In a decentralized healthcare system, where care is provided in more appropriate but more numerous settings, the question of who is responsible for the patient will become a thousand times more sticky. As long as a patient was in one hospital, or was cared for by one physician, there was some hope for coordination of care.

In a new, more fragmented system, who will be the overall protector of the patient? The patient-provider relationship is being recast, but this does not mean that patients should end up having no ongoing relationship with providers. Our best models will likely be found in managed care, along the lines of the "gatekeeper." However, I am not talking about someone who is responsible for the overall financial aspects of a patient's care; I am talking about someone who will be the patient's ethics counselor and advocate.

Another way to approach this is to develop ethics programs in most healthcare settings, not just hospitals and nursing homes. The outpatient or home healthcare or sheltered-housing ethics counselor should be part of the new system.

When Should We Call It Quits?

This will be, in some ways, an extension of what has gone before: When is it time to say enough is enough and terminate treatment?

However, I expect a few new wrinkles. We will be forced to confront situations in which a patient demands continued treatment, even though it is useless, and counseling fails. Providers may have to learn to say "no" in this and other more difficult situations. Also, euthanasia, either passive or active, will again raise its head, as we continue to prolong existence without quality of life.

Patients who want provider help in committing suicide will pose unanswerable questions. And, given the abysmal events of the Eighties, it is inevitable that some of these questions will become legal and political issues—even appearing on ballots—which should do wonders to muddy the waters even further. As Professor Leonard Glantz of Boston University has observed, we may have entered the era of "biological McCarthyism."

What Is Healthcare's Proper Share of the Pie?

Perhaps the toughest issue of all will be determining healthcare's appropriate place in the hierarchy of social needs. During the Eighties, healthcare spending increased 111 percent—while access to care actually decreased. Our sector is already consuming a very large part of the pie—more than 11 percent of the gross national product—and promises to keep on chomping.

What we are buying with these billions of dollars is an interesting question, given our failure in areas such as infant mortality, drug use, child abuse, and mental health. Healthcare will have to engage in some introspection regarding how many resources it deserves in light of other needs—education, rebuilding the infrastructure, protecting the environment, food, and housing—that have gone unmet in recent years.

Healthcare's Teflon is flaking off in terms of its ability to endlessly consume public resources. Current lists of key political and consumer issues do not include healthcare, with the exception of the hot issue of access.

We may have outlived our welcome at the head of the public trough. I, for one, am hard put to defend unbridled proliferation of radiological exotica while hungry children suffer on our streets. In the face of so much preventable suffering, we must take a long look at what we are contributing to ending it, and at what price.

Does all this seem depressing? It isn't. It just has to do with change. A few years ago, polio and pneumonia seemed unstoppable, patients were railroaded by providers who would not listen to them, black Americans had no hope of obtaining even emergency care in many hospitals, and women were barred from becoming doctors or hospital administrators. We had a glut of nurses and few physicians. Some clinical research was conducted with arrogance and deceit, without patient consent or protections.

All that changed, because it had to. And as these new questions emerge, we will find the answers we need—and we will find them, as always, within ourselves.

Out of the Frying Pan . . .

July 1990

I was just one of many people who opposed Oregon's attempt to stretch Medicaid dollars by reducing the services available to low-income Medicaid beneficiaries. The fight went on for a long time; the Bush Administration refused to grant Oregon the necessary waivers, citing discrimination against the disabled (but somehow overlooking the discrimination against the poor). The Clinton Administration granted the waiver, and the program was implemented—in part. The good news is that many more people got healthcare coverage, and, in practice, many (but not all) providers and plans ignored the limitations on services and gave these patients what they needed. The bad news is that the state never got around to implementing universal access, which was doomed by Congressional recalcitrance and Oregon's internal politics. The author of the program, emergency physician John Kitzhaber, was elected governor of Oregon in 1994. I am told that, although the state promised not to do so, it subsequently removed more procedures from the list of what is covered.

R ecently there has been enormous interest in a series of legislative initiatives in Oregon designed, ostensibly, to increase access to healthcare for the poor by limiting the amount of health services available to them, thus stretching public dollars further. The program has been hailed as a real innovation, a step forward in the pursuit of ethical distribution of resources, and a model for other states. From ethicists, legislators, analysts, news media, and providers alike have come roars of approval.

I wish to add my voice to the decidedly smaller chorus of those who are not so enthusiastic—who, in fact, believe that what has been proposed in Oregon violates some of the most basic ethical principles of healthcare.

Setting Priorities?

This all got started several years ago when one of the community ethics projects about which I have written in the past, Oregon Health Decisions, began holding community meetings about how healthcare resources should be distributed. There was widespread consensus that there should be priorities in health services, that is, that some services are more useful and needed than others; that immunization is more valuable than, say, liposuction.

At the same time, the issue of organ transplantation became highly charged in Oregon when a young transplant candidate was denied Medicaid coverage for the procedure, and subsequently died. Again, a question of priorities.

These events had a profound effect on John Kitzhaber, MD (R-Roseburg), the state senate president and an emergency physician, who was involved in Oregon Health Decisions. He began arguing for the setting of priorities to determine which services should be available under Medicaid, and to whom. He also wished to extend Medicaid coverage to more people. In 1989, he submitted legislation codifying this approach, the Oregon Basic Health Services Act. It passed and was signed into law.

It is a package of three bills. The first, S.B. 27, expanded Medicaid eligibility in Oregon from 58 percent of poverty to 100 percent. It also created a system of "prioritization" of health services, so that only those services the legislature is willing to fund will be covered, based on a list developed by a commission and priced by an independent actuary. These priorities are supposed to be developed on the basis of "social values," clinical effectiveness, outcomes, and other criteria.

Also, in a move that was inevitable but raises deeply troubling questions in and of itself, providers are exempted by this legislation from any legal liability for refusing to provide an uncovered service to a Medicaid patient. Regardless of what the effect on the patient might be, hospitals and physicians can now refuse to provide an unreimbursed service with impunity.

This limiting of covered services to a select few will only affect one part of the Medicaid population, however: welfare mothers and children. The elderly, disabled, blind, and long-term care patients will be exempted, despite the fact that these populations consume three-quarters of all Medicaid funds.

The second bill, S.B. 935, mandates that the "basic health benefits package" that emerges from this process be offered by every employer by 1994, so all Oregonians have access to at least the same limited services that the poor have been allotted. This will supposedly cover every working Oregonian with an income at or above poverty level.

Senate Bill 534 creates an insurance pool for coverage of persons deemed "uninsurable" because of poor health status, as other states have done. Although I disapprove of states allowing private insurers to skim healthy candidates while relegating the very sick to the public sector, these pools do provide coverage (although pricey) to the "uninsurable" middle class, and are not the subject of this column.

Legal Obstacles

The prioritization program was to go into effect this summer, but has been stalled because its implementation requires federal waivers that have not been forthcoming. The stripping away of services from Medicaid violates federal law (which mandates that most needed services be provided to Medicaid clients). Congress has been unwilling to grant a waiver, and Oregon has now approached the Health Care Financing Administration in the hope of receiving a warmer welcome there.

The plan to require every employer to provide at least the basic benefits package to workers isn't legal, either. The federal Employee Retirement Income and Security Act (ERISA) prohibits any state except Hawaii (which has a waiver) from regulating the insurance practices of self-insured employers. Oregon can't make self-insured employers provide any coverage, let alone a state-defined package of benefits; thus it cannot guarantee that all employees will be covered. And if Massachusetts, which has been trying for some time to implement universal coverage, has not been able to wangle an ERISA waiver, I doubt that Oregon will.

So although the erosion of Medicaid may be accomplished, the extension of even this stripped-down coverage to all Oregonians likely will not, making it highly questionable that this initiative really constitutes a program of universal access to care.

Making Things Explicit

The rationale offered by Dr. Kitzhaber for this approach includes the argument that rationing has been taking place implicitly and needs to take place explicitly. He also contends that rationing by restricting the availability of care is better than rationing by ability to pay.

These arguments have persuaded many people in healthcare that this is a model answer to the dilemma of restricted resources. Here, they say, is accountability. Here, they say, is an acknowledgment that rationing of healthcare is necessary. Here, they say, is true fairness.

Unfortunately, I don't think it's fair, I don't think it guarantees accountability, and I don't think it achieves anything except diminished access to care for very vulnerable people.

Two Wrongs Don't Make a Right

The most serious problem is the moral flaw that underlies the entire proposal: *It denies care only to the politically powerless poor.* The privately insured can go on getting their liposuctions and carotid endarterectomies and cesarean sections and whatever else they want; this program won't touch them.

No one on Medicare will be affected. Even within the Medicaid population, the blind, disabled, and low-income elderly won't be touched. Just women and children—as usual.

There's Rationing, and Then There's Rationing

There is no question that healthcare is rationed in the United States on the basis of the ability to pay. But does this plan really change that? Kitzhaber is quoted in the November/December 1989 *Hospital Ethics* as saying, "There's nothing to say we can't fund everything for everybody if we want to raise taxes or take money away from schools or corrections." But it is unlikely in the extreme that the legislature will do that.

And as long as most people in Oregon can buy their way into full access to care, it appears that this continues the tradition of rationing by ability to pay. By finding a different way to ration care on that basis, we are not solving the problem. Replacing one unfair rationing scheme with another unfair rationing scheme is not progress.

No Objective Criteria

I believe fervently that any health service's effectiveness, cost-benefit, and appropriateness must be at the forefront of the decision to treat. The known outcomes of a treatment must be the key criteria for its use or denial. If I actually thought this program had the patient experience information, outcomes, and clinical knowledge base to determine what works and what doesn't, and would cover or not cover services on that basis, I would support at least that part of it.

But the development of objective criteria for judging the usefulness of a service is an infant science; at this time, neither the data, nor methodologies, nor the analytical capacity exist except in a few incomplete instances. Rationing on the basis of scientific objectivity is not yet possible. So subjective criteria will prevail.

What will that mean? When kidney dialysis was in very short supply in the 1960s, some research centers tried to evaluate the "social worth" of candidates in order to determine who would have access to the life-saving technology. That process proved to disproportionately favor white, employed, middle-class, married men with children, especially those who attended church and were involved in Boy Scouts.

Could not the same thing happen again? The Oregon health commission's first draft gave the lowest priority to treatment of most conditions associated with AIDS, despite the fact that new treatments are extending the lives of such patients considerably, with good quality of life. Is it the idea of supposedly terminal illness, or the "worthiness" of people with this particular illness, that governed the decision to dismiss their needs?

Also, why must entire classes of services—heart transplants or suicide prevention or other treatments—be denied to all low-income mothers and children? Would it not be better to deny them only in those instances when such care is inadvisable?

Enormous amounts of money could be saved if we provided *only* appropriate care to *all* individuals. And if a treatment is marginal or useless or not indicated, why should it be denied only to the poor? Why should unnecessary or marginal care be available to anyone in Oregon, especially when the legislature has taken the stand that there is not enough money to provide even necessary care to the poor?

Supporting the Status Quo

I fear that this program, far from being an innovation, is actually an attempt to preserve the status quo. It makes no effort to control provider incomes, redirect healthcare spending, or enact reforms to prevent waste. It ignores the question of whether the legislature or the electorate are simply spending too little on healthcare, *and* schools, *and* corrections, in order to retain disposable income.

What has been overlooked, in fact, is that Congress has required *all* states to provide Medicaid coverage to pregnant women and young children with incomes up to 133 percent of the federal poverty line. Oregon's grand gesture appears to be an attempt to fund this Medicaid expansion without raising taxes or looking at other programs' share of the pie.

Also, there is no guarantee that providers will care for patients who are supposedly covered. Physicians (and, one presumes, the now-indemnified hospitals) are free to pick and choose whom they will treat. In these days of skimpy provider payments and discriminatory patient selection, coverage is no longer any guarantee of access.

As Robert Sillen, executive director of Santa Clara Valley Medical Center, has said, "Last time I looked, Medicaid was an insurance program. Yet there are many places in this country where a pregnant woman on Medicaid can't get anyone to deliver her baby, let alone give her prenatal care!" What guarantees that the few services that *are* funded will really be available to Medicaid patients in Oregon?

How Much Democracy?

Senator Orrin Hatch (R-UT), who is hardly known for espousing universal access, has been quoted as saying that the Oregon proposal is so impressive that "we should get together the finest minds on biomedical ethics, public health, and medical economics. They should consult with the American Medical Association, Medicare officials, and other responsible organizations in the field, and draw up a set of guidelines."

While these healthcare leaders decide who should get what, perhaps they could consult the one group noticeably absent from Hatch's list: the patients who will suffer as a result of the choices made by all these heavy hitters.

I have long believed that one element critical to the making of ethical policy is that *the people who will bear the brunt of policy choices should have some say in those choices*. The people of Seward, Alaska, as the oil from the *Exxon Valdez* swirled toward them, held a town meeting to decide which parts of the area should be saved with the booms they had. They chose to save the salmon streams and not the wild bays; the mayor later said that it might not have been the right choice, but it was *their* choice, and they were the ones who would have to live with it.

Of the thousands of Oregonians who participated in the Oregon Health Decisions community meetings, how many were children and low-income mothers? And how many of the people at those meetings knew that their call for prioritization would be translated into denial of the poor?

There will supposedly be four "consumers" on the health commission; none will be children. None will be the inarticulate, the non-English-speaking, the illiterate, the chronically ill, the frightened, the depressed, the beaten-down. Even if they are, they can always be voted down by the other seven members. Not one member of the Oregon legislature, I'll wager, is on Medicaid, ever has been on Medicaid, or ever will be. They are not liable to the rationing they are so blithely laying on the poorest of the poor.

James Tallon, Jr. (D-Binghamton), the majority leader of the New York State Assembly, has spoken eloquently on this point: "If we are all subject to the question, then it is legitimate for society to ask it. If we are not all included, then it is an illegitimate question, because we have not established the ethical baseline of all of us being at equal risk simultaneously."

I agree; if access to care will be restricted to a few services, then everyone—including the members of the Oregon legislature—should face the same restrictions.

Making decisions that we know will not affect us creates an unforgivable callousness of policy, and erects an unconscionable barrier between us and the consequences of our decisions.

The Day May Come

It is entirely possible that, driven by the dreadful increase in health-care spending, the legacy of years of disdain for the poor and the different, and the fuzziness of mission that has come to characterize so much of healthcare, this plan will be implemented—and imitated. Thus the health economy could be formalized in two sectors: one wasteful, self-indulgent, and wealthy, and the other something out of the Third World.

Should that happen, the price paid by society as a whole could well exceed the price paid by the victims. For meanness, whether intentional or not, is toxic beyond measure. The English mystery writer P.D. James, when asked why her murder tales are so grim and hopeless, responded, "Murder is a really contaminating crime, and no life that comes in touch with it remains unaltered. In the end, the murder may be solved, but justice hasn't necessarily been done."

In the end, the Oregon legislature and its supporters may win the short-term battle, keeping access and taxes both fashionably low; but the price of that convenience may be more than a civilized society should be willing to pay.

Doing It Yourself

September 1990

Some topics in bioethics inspire reasoned debate, such as the proper patient-provider relationship. Some ethics topics produce passionate discourse, such as abortion. And some ethics topics produce cold chills in everyone. Such a topic is suicide by patients.

I have a very complicated view of suicide, and it has its roots in a number of factors. First, people close to me have taken their own lives, and I have been hurt by their actions, so it is a matter of great sensitivity for me.

Second, there are different kinds of suicide, ranging from attempts to draw the attention of others to desperate acts by those who believe that life is no longer worthwhile. Some are a response to terrible pain. Some are the expression of a desire by a dying person to retain control over the circumstances of his or her death.

Some suicides are planned; others are spur-of-the-moment. Some are acts of vengeance directed at others, whereas others are inner-directed. Some people who kill themselves are in full control of their faculties; others do not know what they are doing, and may not mean to die.

Third, although there is a rich religious literature on suicide, I think about ethics in secular terms. And because there are strong religious doctrines concerning suicide (pro and con), I do not wish to offend those with deeply held religious beliefs.

Nevertheless, there has been so much discussion about the issue lately that I wanted to offer some thoughts. These are personal views, stated in secular terms, and are offered mainly as starting points for discussion. In this as in so many areas of ethics, I do not believe there are absolute answers out there waiting for us to uncover them.

Is Suicide Ever Justifiable?

In that suicide involves the taking of human life, many people say it is never justified. However, I am reminded of a statement made to me once by a psychiatrist. I came to interview him for a story the day after a patient of his had committed suicide by leaping from a building. I offered my condolences, and he said, "People fail to understand that some mental illness is terminal."

I have pondered his words many times. And, having seen the results of profound depression in people, I can understand how that toxic disease could lead inevitably to suicide.

Not enough of us understand that severe mental pain can be just as awful as severe physical pain—in some cases more so, because treatment and palliation can be harder to come by. When we hear of the suicide of an individual suffering from a physical disease— Ernest Hemingway shooting himself rather than undergo the last painful stages of cancer, for example—we understand the act.

But when the great psychiatrist Bruno Bettelheim commits suicide because of apparently great mental pain, we are more puzzled. Perhaps it is that more of us have suffered great physical pain than have suffered great mental pain, and therefore do not know how devastating it can be.

We also tend to distinguish between the suicide of someone who is profoundly or terminally ill, and the suicide of someone not so afflicted. And we mourn the suicide of the young more than that of someone of advanced years. These are social judgments more than clinical ones, and they may not stand up well under scrutiny; yet they influence whether we see suicide as justified.

Suicide may not be a rational act, but I think it can be justified. In many instances it is probably or absolutely the best of a set of terrible choices, and therefore should not be condemned out of hand. But it must always be treated as the most extreme of acts—and should not be condoned by others without utterly compelling reason.

I have grieved when people about whom I cared committed suicide, especially in those cases when I did not believe it was the best option. But I do think each of us is the owner of his or her life, and can thus end it. Governments, providers, religions, or other entities that claim they have a greater claim to my life than I do are violating the most basic of all principles of liberty.

Should Providers Prevent Suicide?

Providers have an ethical duty to consider a patient's wish for suicide very carefully and to intervene when that wish seems misguided, based on the individual circumstances of the patient. I specifically exclude situations when a provider's religious beliefs, such as the conviction that all suicide is wrong, prevent that provider from considering the individual patient's situation. As my beliefs are based on the rights of the individual patient, across-the-board religious doctrine cannot be a criterion for intervention because it is not a response to an individual circumstance.

Still, too many of us, in our zeal to honor patients' rights, ignore both the proper role of paternalism in the patient-provider relationship and the strong possibility that the patient may be wrong in choosing suicide.

I was most heavily influenced on this point by a classic article: "Patient Autonomy and 'Death with Dignity,'" by David L. Jackson and Stuart Youngner, which appeared originally in the August 23, 1979 *New England Journal of Medicine*. The authors argue brilliantly that providers' preoccupation with honoring patients' rights might affect their clinical judgment and lead them to ignore factors that could produce an inappropriate wish to die: patient ambivalence, depression, an unexpressed problem, fear of further treatment, differences in family and patient perception of the situation, and staff misconceptions about the patient's stated wish for death.

Although many of these issues come up in discussions of termination of treatment for the terminally ill, I do not think we take them seriously enough when a patient is considering suicide. Depression, especially, is a silent epidemic, particularly prevalent and untreated among the elderly and the poor.

How much attention do we pay to talk of suicide by an old woman in pain from chronic arthritis, who is lonely and depressed? Too often we view her suicide as inevitable—or even appropriate. We are hardly as philosophical about the suicides of teenagers. Providers' attitudes toward patient suicide are inevitably influenced by provider values; we must strive for greater consistency and valuing of all patients.

Should Providers Abet the Suicide of Patients?

Fine distinctions darken the already muddy waters of this issue. Is the patient terminally ill and/or in agony? Is the patient capable of suicide without the provider's help? Is it abetting the act to not report the suicidal intentions of a patient?

Is it suicide or murder when, at a patient's request, a physician administers a lethal dose of drugs, as in the case reported anonymously in the notorious "Debbie" commentary in the *Journal of the American Medical Association* (January 8, 1988)? What if the drugs are just left at the bedside or with the family?

I believe there are times when a provider can ethically aid in a suicide—there are even times when it may even appear necessary— but they are few and far between. When Jack Kevorkian, MD, made the headlines with his "suicide machine" in Michigan, and public opinion surveys showed a majority of Americans believed he and Janet Adkins, whose death he abetted (or caused), had the right to do what they did, I was deeply troubled. I was not distressed by the patient's decision: if she felt it was best to take her life, then I believe she had that right.

It was Kevorkian's role that bothered me. During the "Debbie" furor, a consistent criticism of the physician who administered the lethal dose of drugs was that he had never seen the patient before. I think that is an extremely important point, and it applies here as well.

To aid a suicide is as serious an act as a caregiver can undertake; it should never be undertaken by a provider who does not know the patient well. Otherwise we dehumanize patient and provider alike. We also cheapen life by taking it lightly, which is what eventually led to the mass euthanasia and genocide of Nazi medicine.

I also do not believe that a provider should abet a suicide for profit or for pay of any kind, even to "cover expenses." I hardly think this needs to be explained.

Nor do I think that provider aiding of patient suicide should be decriminalized. I cannot be so sure about indemnification of providers against malpractice litigation in such cases. The malpractice situation has become such a swamp that I find it easy to believe that a physician could aid a patient's suicide only to be sued by the patient's family, or could aid an unsuccessful suicide and be sued for blowing the job.

I oppose decriminalizing the aiding of suicide for three reasons: (1) I do not think suicide should ever be made easy; (2) I do not think that providers are so free of bias and emotion that they will always make the right decision when a patient asks for help in ending his or her life, and there thus must be some accountability; and (3) I know that most provider-abetted suicides—and they take place every day—are the result of a private, profoundly considered covenant between the patient and the provider.

That is probably as it should be. Because suicide, on some level, is an antisocial act—even if I do believe it to be a right—then society should not sanction it freely. It is best kept a private affair, undertaken with caution.

Should Providers Be Forced to Abet a Suicide?

Never. Several years ago, Elizabeth Bouvia sought to force a hospital to allow her to starve to death as a patient there. At the time, George Annas of Boston University and I got into a lively public discussion of whether Bouvia was within her rights.

I argued that she was not. He believed she was, in part because there was no place in the healthcare system for someone like Elizabeth Bouvia to face life and death on her own terms. She was too physically incapacitated to carry out her own wishes.

Indeed, healthcare had no place for her; but that was not the point. Simply because a patient seeks death does not mean caregivers should be forced to abet that patient's suicide. It violates the primary commitment of most physicians, nurses, social workers, and other providers. *Voluntary* participation in a suicide is an individual choice; *forced* participation is a violation of provider rights as destructive as denial of patients' rights.

The issue of suicide will keep coming back to us, more forcefully every time. I think the healthcare field, by and large, is unprepared to deal with many of the questions it raises. I hope we will address them before we are forced to by public opinion and the pressure of events.

Is It Worth It?

November 1990

A physician who is a "high admitter" to the hospital and a major source of revenue is also a danger to patients—an incompetent surgeon who performs unnecessary procedures to boot. Some medical staff physicians want to demand that his privileges be withdrawn, but they fear that the hospital will do nothing—and that they are risking a lawsuit.

A nurse witnesses a clear instance of malpractice on the part of a physician and wants to tell the quality assurance committees of the board and medical staff. She is warned off by colleagues who tell her that in such situations, the nurse is the one who ends up getting punished.

Family members, despondent over the persistent vegetative state into which their relative has fallen, beg the hospital chaplain to intervene with hospital authorities who are refusing to allow life support to be discontinued for legal reasons. The chaplain is concerned that his doing so might compromise his role as a neutral counselor and arbiter—and anger the administration.

An emergency department physician wants to admit an indigent uninsured patient who is not in a life-threatening condition but needs treatment so that her condition does not deteriorate further. The administrator reminds the physician that the hospital, wealthy as it is, has a policy of refusing to admit the uninsured except when they are in extremis. The

physician says she may go to the press—and is threatened with
revocation of her privileges.

. . . .

These stories, unfortunately, may have a familiar ring. They have all happened. In talking with the people who told me about them, I was asked the same question each time: "Why take the risk? Is it worth it?"

It's a good question—and one that some bioethicists find threatening. There are reasons for that. Bioethics is top-heavy with theoreticians who hold conferences and explain things to each other. Too often, their base is theoretical, their experience minimal, and their contact with practitioners nonexistent.

As a result, they can create other-worldly models of great eloquence and style that are of little or no use to the night shift at Memorial Hospital. It is easy for a bioethics type with a tenured academic appointment to tell a healthcare worker to risk his or her job in order to right a wrong.

Also, most of us—I daresay virtually all of us—would like to live in a world in which the choices are clear between right and wrong, we are always on the side of the angels, the good guys always win, and nobody gets hurt. In such a world, which is the world for which too much bioethical philosophy is developed, risk-taking is not really risky because Right Always Triumphs.

Too bad that the real situation is more likely to be that of a nurse who is the sole support of two young children and who has finally landed a job with guaranteed shifts and good benefits. Maybe she has a mortgage as well. And she fears that if she turns in Doctor Jones, she is more likely to be censured—perhaps even dismissed—than she is to achieve the protection of patients against the good doctor.

Well, if she's a nurse, you say, she can get another job easily. Maybe, but it might not be as good a job. Maybe she *likes* her job. And what if she is a low-echelon housekeeper or security guard?

Issues of accountability, risk-taking, and courage can be very ugly in the practice setting. We may be willing to take a risk, even a big risk, but what do we do if we think the chain of command may not back us? If there is cowardice between us and what we need to do, why should we take risks that will surely amount to nothing?

There is no simple answer, but there are ways to judge the quality of a risk and the necessity of taking it. Keep in mind that my perspective is unusual: I can take more risks than some people. I have neither children nor mortgage, and therefore am not as constrained as are those who do.

Furthermore, I am self-employed; I may starve next year for lack of work, but I do not have a salaried job to lose. I live with this fragile arrangement precisely because I want to be able to speak my mind, even though this kind of life has prices of its own.

The factors that go into my consideration of risk are different in some ways than the factors affecting those with family responsibilities. As I recently told a friend who was considering a move that could endanger his child's future, "If you're going to gamble, you should probably do it only with your own money, not with that of those who depend on you."

So: If you must take a risk in order to achieve an ethical good, how do you judge the relative consequences of doing it or not doing it?

Are You Alone?

The most dicey situation is if you think you have no allies. That, in itself, is reason to consider carefully if this is something you really feel you must do. If no one is standing with you, there may be a good reason; perhaps you should reconsider. In any case, it is important to seek allies. There is a geometric increase in the strength of your position if more people share it.

Discovering or developing allies also can provide you with more ammunition, better strategy, logistical and emotional support, and protection against fear. However, if you have to go it alone, then go it alone. When we cease believing that one person can have an impact, we have lost the ethical basis of democracy.

Where Do You Present the Problem?

A good way to foul up the presentation of an ethical problem is to tell it to the wrong person and/or in the wrong place. That is why ethics committees have proven to be such a godsend. A good ethics committee should be open to any sincerely felt ethical problem—and should deal with it in confidence.

In my experience with ethics committees, however, I have found that they are much more comfortable dealing with problems involving termination of treatment and family issues than with accusations against the chief of surgery.

Nevertheless, if there is an ethics committee, it should probably be your first stop. (If the problem involves someone who sits on the ethics committee—and that has been known to happen—ask for a private meeting with the chairperson or vice-chairperson of the committee.)

Also, there may be a board member, or a manager outside your chain of command, whom you see as fair. Approach him or her if your own hierarchy is unapproachable, or if you perceive it to be so, or if there is a conflict of interest involved. However, be warned that in any organization, those in leadership positions prefer that normal procedure be followed: Be prepared to present a strong enough case to justify your having gone outside normal channels.

What Are the Stakes?

This simply means that you should pick your fights. If someone took a long lunch hour and logged it as work, it's irritating and worthy of mention to the offender, but it's hardly worth starting a war. But if patients are in danger, or if a fellow worker is at risk unjustifiably, then the stakes are high indeed, and your duty is clearer.

Everyone in healthcare—even those of us on its fringes—has a paramount duty to protect patients, beyond anything else, even fiduciary responsibilities or professional collegiality. Abandoning patients is the cardinal sin; they are always worth the risk. Remember, they aren't patients because they want to be; they are forced to trust us.

This is perhaps the most difficult question, because the stakes include not only you and whoever else is involved, but also your family, others who may depend on you, and your role in the organization. It is not selfish to consider these things; wanting to be a good provider is an honorable goal that is worth pursuing. If you have helped patients and have protected them against harm, then you should consider the consequences of your being transferred, dismissed, or involved in long, hairy litigation.

Milton wrote, after going blind, "They also serve who only stand and wait." I believe that—strongly enough that I generally think that if there is a way by which you can stick around and continue to be of service, you should.

Sometimes, however, that is not possible.

What If It Seems Hopeless?

I was in San Antonio earlier this year, which gave me the chance to revisit the Alamo, something of a cultural icon in my family (my mother was a devout Texan). As I walked around the old mission, I was struck by the reverence in which we hold a highly romantic but doomed gesture on the part of men who may well have been of more use had they managed to survive. We honor their memory, but some of us question their sense.

Still, there are times when you must make a stand and take the consequences, even if you fear you will not win. If to do otherwise is cowardly and unethical, you have to play Davy Crockett. It is a very personal decision and can be easily second-guessed.

I was once elected to the employee relations committee of a firm I worked for. We received complaints from minority workers about hiring and promotion policies and unequal pay. The committee asked a task force, led by me, to check it out. The firm refused our requests for even basic data, and told us to mind our own business.

I felt I had to resign, and did. I might well have been able to do more if I had stayed on the committee, but I felt that I could not do so in good conscience. We all have our Alamos; they all have their prices.

How Do You Deal with the Fear?

Fear can be either a good warning or a paper tiger. To the degree that it inspires reasonable caution, we should respect it; there's a good reason we are afraid to jump off five-story buildings. To the degree that fear provides us with an excuse for copping out, we have to brush it aside. If the risk has to be taken, it has to be taken; fear cannot win instead. Most of us are adults, which means we are responsible for the consequences of our actions—and inaction.

In our youth, we were taught to obey the rules and to fear punishment. Generally, that's good advice. And fortunately, healthcare is starting to provide protection to those who challenge ethical wrongs. But it will be a while before these mechanisms are universal. In the meantime, we cannot abandon duty because we are afraid of a spanking.

The Ethics of Advocacy and Policy
Honor Among Thieves?

January 1991

The new Congress has been seated. Many state legislatures are in session. Healthcare, as a big consumer of public money (it is, along with education, one of the two biggest consumers of state money), will be under scrutiny by all levels of government. International events, the savings and loan mess, a shaky economy, and federal and state budget deficits will likely force limitations in public funding for health services.

All this guarantees yet another re-examination of health policy, which means fervent efforts by healthcare lobbyists—professional and amateur—to direct the shape of policy reform.

For many, this will be an exercise in cynicism, measured in favors and funds. For others, it will be an exercise in sheer power. But for some—lobbyists and legislators alike—it could also be an exercise in ethics. There *are* honorable ways to make and influence health policy.

You may think that ethics and policymaking are not compatible—that, in fact, ethical policymaking is a contradiction in terms. I do not believe that is true.

It's easy to disparage politicians and the political process; too often, they give us ample reason to disparage them. But we must be doing something right politically. We are the oldest continuous democracy in the world, and folks in Chile, Haiti, Eastern Europe, and other places want to join the party.

Democracy is messy, confusing, time-consuming, driven too much by economics, riddled with special interests, wildly inefficient, and too often hands you a poodle when you were hoping for a camel. But to paraphrase Winston Churchill, it beats the alternatives.

So, in the spirit of ethical lobbying and moral policymaking, here are six principles to keep in mind when you are in the political trenches, seeking to shape the future of American healthcare.

1. Choose your causes wisely. Obviously, whenever health legislation or regulations are proposed, healthcare professionals must be aware of them and respond when necessary. But it is unwise to start World War III over every single proposal. And it is particularly fruitless to oppose, with your dying breath, something that is going to pass regardless of what you do (except in those cases where an issue of paramount moral significance is involved).

So don't spend all your time coiled in place, ready to pounce. Always seek cooperation and accommodation first. Try to be a friend of the policy process.

We are taught from an early age that Americans are supposed to be rugged individualists, striding against the tide, alone on the mountain (it's a high tide), standing up for our principles, never giving up or giving in. This mythic stance is a luxury that policy can rarely afford.

Don't waste moral capital, which is even more precious than political capital, by engaging in petty or unimportant fights over details. Go to war only when you must, and when your reasons for thinking you must will appear justified under the harshest of press and public scrutiny.

2. Don't accept apparent limits unless you know they are real. Drew Altman, president of the Henry J. Kaiser Family Foundation in California, who also served as commissioner of the Department of Human Services for the state of New Jersey for several years, once said this is the most important point in advocating for fair policy.

He thought that if he had fought just a bit harder for some things he believed in, he would have won.

Therefore, we must seek to determine if the limits that are thrown up to us are real. I have often told the story about an incident in Brazil in 1985, when prison overcrowding became so horrendous that the inmates in some prisons took matters into their own hands. They cast lots in certain cell blocks, and hanged the losers. Although we recoil from this solution, it's important to understand why we do so.

In theory, it has a lot of good points: It is democratic, it is self-imposed by those involved, it creates the benefit of more room, and it uses an objective means of selection. It seems to fit the requirements of theoretical ethics. So why does it trouble us?

It makes us cringe because the inmates assumed they had no choice but to commit murder—however democratically—while we on the outside know there were many other and less brutal options, from parole and probation to building more prisons, inaugurating work-release programs, setting up cots in the parking lot, reducing sentences, or other alternatives.

But the inmates in Brazil could not see beyond the limits of their own situation, and no one else cared enough to intervene and stretch those limits, so the inmates felt they had no choice but to kill each other.

In making policy, *apparent* limits are too often seen as engraved in stone. Yet there is a tremendous capacity for flexibility in policymaking. New York and California, and, to a lesser degree, Texas and Florida, have found funds—not enough, but some—to treat the victims of a sudden and vicious epidemic that has largely victimized unpopular social groups.

States are coping with mandated increases in Medicaid eligibility. There are many programs seeking to preserve and even enhance rural healthcare services. And several states are sincerely pursuing the goal of universal access to care for all their residents.

Innovation is alive and well, and will continue to be, as long as the essential ingredient is there: a belief that most limits can be challenged. And foremost among the limits that must be challenged is the belief that the poorer and more powerless you are, the less you deserve the government's attention. Health policy has foundered on this shoal more than on any other.

Government pampering of the privileged, which reached ridiculous levels in the Eighties, is starting to produce a backlash. Policymakers and lobbyists can take advantage of that reaction to move back in the direction of honesty and justice. Insurance regulation, Medicaid configurations, commitment to public health, differentiation between fat and sassy hospitals and those that are hanging on by their fingernails, and the false assumption that a heartless nation will not spend any more money on the helpless—these are the areas in which we need to change the alleged rules.

It boils down to the ethical responsibility of government. There are many who say that the primary duty of government is to self-destruct. It is this ethic (such as it is) that in recent years has led us to elect people who hate government, who often see it simply as a means of personal enrichment.

But there are others—myself included—who believe that government has at least three primary ethical responsibilities. One is to husband public resources rather than rifle them. Another is to be a voice, a surrogate, for those who have no power and no voice. And a third is to reallocate resources so that a basic level of equity is available to all. How you define the limits of health policy depends on which definition of government duty you embrace.

3. Give those most affected by policy decisions some voice in those choices. Although one of the principles of democracy is that we elect people to represent us who will express our views by proxy, that is not always how it happens. Ours is an enclave society; we tend to live with, work with, and vote for people with whom we feel a cultural, ethnic, or class bond. That can leave a lot of people out of the political power game.

Furthermore, elected officials work within complex webs of power, so they tend to heed the views of the wealthy and influential more than they do the views of the disenfranchised. The transfer of wealth from the poor and near-poor to the rich in the last decade was sorry evidence of this.

Despite these complications, I believe that if you are the one who will pay the price or endure the suffering engendered by policy decisions, you have a right to help determine how that price will be paid or the suffering played out. Too often, those who will bear the burden are excluded from the deliberations.

This is why I become so enraged at polite, elite discussions about "rationing of healthcare" that take place among well-insured upper-class intellectuals who are only interested in rationing care to the uninsured or Medicaid-dependent poor. Medicaid was once described as a program designed by the rich to tax the middle class to protect the poor, and thus was doomed to be an albatross. Although it has survived, it has consistently suffered from the class bias out of which it sprang—as has much health policy since.

So if we want to make ethical policy, we must try to include those who will be most affected. In a democracy, that is the most ethical approach, but it can be monumentally difficult. Even when you get a consensus and everyone agrees to a tough decision, most of them will want to be exempted from the implementation of that decision if it actually becomes applicable to them.

My child always deserves an organ transplant; it's those *other* families who are being selfish, gaming the system, and misusing the transplant resource.

Nevertheless, if people are to be made to suffer, they deserve a shot at helping determine how they will suffer.

4. Recognize that some changes take a long time. This is a nation of instant gratification, from fast food to automatic teller machines. We don't want to wait. This is why we condemn queuing for health services in other countries, calling it unacceptable rationing, despite the fact that 15 to 20 percent of Americans have no guarantee that they will get *any* healthcare, no matter how long they wait. We want everything now.

Yet patience is a virtue in politics, and the more complex the issue, the more patience is needed. Even Americans can learn patience; the prize is just that much sweeter when it is finally won. (I speak to this from an expert point of view, for I am a fan of the Chicago Cubs.)

In many cases, the most ethical position you can take is to keep pushing, to be one more voice in a chorus that is getting imperceptibly stronger, to move the elephant forward an inch, to talk even one more person into joining the fight.

That is how we make policy in this country, in an endless bunny hop of 100 steps forward and 99 back again. Every single one of those steps is important, not just numbers 1 and 100. (Although the Cubs last won a World Series 39 years before I was born, I am not without hope. Wait 'til next year!)

Because healthcare, and the policies that direct it, change so slowly and reluctantly, it is especially important that we learn to commit for the long run. In a television movie about the efforts of the Walsh family of Florida, whose son was kidnaped and murdered, to establish a federal system of quick response in such situations, the father is disheartened after he has testified yet again before Congress, seemingly to no avail.

He asks a congressional staffer, "How long do you have to keep saying these things?" The man replies: "As long as it takes."

5. Work for the public accountability of those who make the decisions. I once asked Robert Blendon, now chairman of the Department of Health Policy and Management at the Harvard School of Public Health, if he thought we should have an integrated national healthcare database.

He said he would not support any data system so big and cumbersome that it would make data available five years after the fact. As it is now, he said, most officials are out of office by the time the results of their handiwork become evident. Their accountability is thus nonexistent.

It is morally necessary, especially when decisions are difficult and their consequences grave, that the people who make the decisions are known to the public and judged by the public, in order to ensure their accountability. Political figures are supposed to be publicly accountable, of course, but too much of what they do seems to take place in the dark, away from public view.

When the options dwindle and things get tight, the best chance for a socially responsible, ethical solution is to get decisionmaking out of the back room and into the light. I believe that public scrutiny contributes immeasurably to the ethical behavior of decisionmakers because public accountability, sooner or later, tends to force higher ethical standards.

Not always. The electorate loses its mind from time to time and is swayed by the most base and despicable arguments. But the ship of state always rights itself—in time.

We are better off seeking a higher moral standard of policymaking, even if we don't always succeed, than we are pandering to hatred, ignorance, and lack of accountability, seeking to cut secret deals rather than cutting the strings that are so often attached to those deals.

6. Exercise vision. There are times, when a wrong is being committed in your name or when you are asked to support or participate in a wrong act, that you have to stand up and say no. And there are times when you have to go out on a limb without the guarantee—perhaps even without the expectation—that the good guys will win. Sometimes, rather than caving in to the expediency of the moment, you have to believe in the future, and try to serve it.

Vision can be a powerful political force, even in the face of bigotry, selfishness, and stupidity. At those times when public opinion favors injustice, it is incumbent upon those in leadership positions to exercise vision and refuse to give in to it; it is simply too late in the history of this republic to allow baseness to dictate policy.

Vision is no guarantee. It can save the day; it can also be a one-way ticket back to Poughkeepsie. Nevertheless, in the end, in difficult times even more than in flush times, it is vision that gets things done. For although Americans are obsessed with superficial beauty, mesmerized by money, and entranced by selfishness, they are more impressed by courage, and will not only forgive it but in time will follow it.

In a nation hungry for inspiration, dispirited by immorality, and frightened of tomorrow, the future belongs to people of vision, courage, and ethical strength—those who know we are all in this together.

It can be a terrible game, this politics. It always has been. But it remains *our* game, uniquely and insanely ours. A great many people have died to keep it so. The least we can do to honor their memory, and our own consciences, is to try to keep a balance in policymaking between pragmatism and honor.

• • • • • • •

This article is based on principles originally developed for presentation at the 1989 meeting of the National Academy for State Health Policy, the 1989 Chicago-Cook County Health Care Summit, and the 1990 California Conference on the Future of Public Health. They have also been presented, in one form or another, at conferences sponsored by the District of Columbia and Minnesota hospital associations.

An Ethic for All of Us

March 1991

A historical note: The Cruzan case involved a young woman, Nancy Cruzan, who was left in a persistent vegetative state by an auto accident. After years of waiting for improvement that did not occur, her parents sought to terminate her hydration and nutrition, which they believed was her wish. The state of Missouri, where she was institutionalized, fought the parents and sought to establish that the state had an overriding interest in "the sanctity of life," which many observers thought had more to do with abortion than with Nancy Cruzan. The U.S. Supreme Court, in a landmark decision, upheld Missouri's claim, but only because the Cruzans had not offered "clear and convincing evidence" that their daughter would have refused nutrition and hydration. In addition, the Court gave guarded support to the validity of living wills as such evidence. A lower court eventually honored the Cruzans' request after they were able to produce witnesses who attested to Nancy Cruzan's wishes. The entire case was highly controversial, and its low point was probably reached when anti-abortion activists tried to break into her room and force-feed her after her parents won their case.

I n thinking about the relationship of ecology to ethics, one's first instinctive thought is that the ecology movement is unimpeachably ethical. What could be more right than protecting trees and flowers and bunnies? What could be more appropriate than health-care professionals—who consider themselves protectors of others—contributing to these efforts?

One's second thought is that all providers have an ethical duty to be ecologically responsible—to recycle materials, to refrain from polluting, to protect the environment. Indeed, healthcare providers might well be expected to hold to a higher ecological standard than others.

When medical waste began washing up on East Coast beaches three years ago, three fears were expressed in the news reports. The first, of course, was that the AIDS virus was being set loose on the land (it wasn't). The second was concern about bathers stepping on needles or being cut by glass or infected by something other than HIV.

The third concern was that hospitals might be responsible for this; this prospect somehow was much worse than if another entity—in this case, probably the Navy or illegal private dumpers—had discarded the waste into the sea.

The involvement of healthcare providers—individual and organizational—in ecological activities is, needless to say, right and proper. However, I don't think the interrelationship of healthcare, ethics, and the environment stops there. Healthcare ethics can learn much from the environmental movement. Among these lessons:

Ethics must be applied on both the "macro" and "micro" level to be effective. One of the most interesting aspects of the ecology movement—and one reason for its success—has been its ability to appeal to both personal desire and the sense of social responsibility. It provides an attractive cause for the individual as an individual as well as for the individual as part of society.

One can argue for recycling on both the individual level (this will make my personal environment more attractive by saving trees and other natural things that I wish to look at) and the social level (in recycling these things, I will reduce the amount of land that must go to landfills, as well as providing jobs and revenue for those who recycle).

However, there are dangers in trying to appeal to both self and selflessness. A sense of individual responsibility can deteriorate into arrogance and judgmentalism, which in turn can overwhelm social concerns. This tension is rife in the environmental movement; some people who started out as nature-loving bunny protectors have become quite intolerant of those who cannot or do not engage in the conservation practices that environmentalists want them to follow.

As we have seen with the anti-smoking movement, what starts out as a desire to improve ends up as a drive to terrorize those of whom we do not approve. We are soon so Machiavellian in our pursuit of what we want that we are willing to violate other people's rights, gloss over complex issues, and condemn those who do not measure up to our standards. A communal movement becomes a hypocritical pogrom.

We run a similar risk in healthcare ethics when we become so focused on the individual aspect of an ethics problem that we neglect the social aspect of that problem. Sometimes we think there is no social aspect. Yet all ethics problems have their social aspects.

Many of us viewed the recent legal fight over Nancy Cruzan's hydration and nutrition to be a straightforward matter of an individual's right not to have her "life" (such as it was) artificially prolonged. Yet the case became entangled in social issues such as a state's interest in the sanctity of life and the national debate over abortion. If their surfaces are scratched, even the most individualized ethics problems prove to have social impacts and considerations.

In a passionate and controversial essay published in 1984, sociologists Rene Fox and Judith Swazey argued, in fact, that bioethics had developed such an individualistic and intellectualized focus that it routinely ignored the social and community aspects of the problems it sought to address.

They wrote: "The emphasis that bioethics places on individualism and on contractual relations freely entered into by voluntarily consenting adults tends to minimize and obscure the interconnectedness of persons and the social and moral importance of their interrelatedness. . . . [This] restricted definition of 'persons as individuals' and 'persons in relations' that pervades bioethics makes it difficult to find an appropriate place for values like decency, kindness, empathy, caring, devotion, service, generosity, altruism, sacrifice, and love. . . .

"Values like these, that center on the bonds between self and others and on community, and that include both 'strangers' and 'brothers,' and future as well as present generations in their orbit, are categorized in bioethics as sociological, theological, or religious rather than as ethical or moral." (Fox, R. and Swazey, J. "Medical Morality Is Not Bioethics: Medical Ethics in China and the United States," *Perspectives in Biology and Medicine*, Vol. 27, No. 3, Spring 1984)

Their argument was roundly criticized at the time; but I think it was accurate and relevant then and is even more so now.

So far—with a few exceptions—the environmental movement has done a far better job of balancing individual and social interests than has healthcare ethics. Bioethics needs to find a middle ground—not only because we are all simultaneously individuals and social beings, but also because we will be more successful if we work from both perspectives, as the environmentalists have done.

An ethic based on rights is not the same as an ethic based on responsibilities. Fox and Swazey also wrote that "the concept and language of 'rights' prevail over those of 'responsibility' and 'obligation' in bioethical discourse, and the term 'duty' does not appear often in the bioethical vocabulary." Indeed, they argued, in American bioethics, "the 'collective good' tends to be seen atomistically and arithmetically as the sum total of the rights and interests, desires, and demands of an aggregate of self-contained individuals." Obligations and responsibilities thus play second fiddle in American healthcare ethics.

The environmental movement has done better than this in accepting obligation and altruism as valid reasons for pursuing conservation goals; one can act unselfishly and not be thought a fool. Many of those who supported protecting the habitats of the snail darter or the northern spotted owl had little expectation that they would ever get to see one of these critters in the field; most of those who wept for Prince William Sound had never seen the place.

The environmental movement uses both the language of rights and the language of responsibility; it has thus given us a lesson in the value and meaning of obligation. If we have a right to a safe and attractive environment, we also have an obligation to protect it.

Whether we exercise that obligation in a small way, by recycling or refraining from littering, or in a large way, by cleaning out littered creeks or washing oil-soaked sea birds, we are not confined to acts of traditional self-interest. One may act out of altruism within the ethic of ecology.

In healthcare, unfortunately, there has been a less even balance between selfishness and service. Bioethics, in its zealous pursuit of rights, has often ignored the concomitant responsibilities those rights entail. The patient's right to know, for example, should not be compromised, but there is a responsibility to honor that right in a way that does not send the patient into a suicidal depression.

The patient's right to informed consent does not mean the provider may discard his or her obligation to counsel, advise, and guide the patient in a shared decisionmaking process. We fuss over the right of an individual patient to terminate treatment but refuse to acknowledge any right of access for uninsured, poor children.

And the fact that service is the basis of healthcare—which is irrefutable, despite all the yammer about "product lines"—does not mean the healthcare system has the right to exploit its workers and volunteers simply because they wish to be of service. The American hospital system was built on the backs of unpaid nurses, whose lives were often little different from those of medieval serfs.

Susan Reverby has written eloquently about the price of caring in such a context, about the dilemma of nurses being "ordered to care in a society that refuses to value caring." (Susan Reverby, *Ordered to Care: The Dilemma of American Nursing, 1850-1945*, Cambridge University Press, 1987) Healthcare has a responsibility to value and reward those who care and serve. Let us again learn from ecology: Rights and responsibilities are equally important.

All ethics are interconnected, because of the fundamental relationship that underlies them. Three years after the Fox and Swazey essay was published, Van Rensselaer Potter of the University of Wisconsin wrote an essay in which he supported much of what Fox and Swazey had said, noting that rampant individualism produces a skewed ethic. He also argued that bioethics is hindered by a narrow tunnel vision that reflects a medical culture beset by the same problem.

He protested the narrow definition of "bioethics" as a subspecialized medical concept that excludes the nonclinical aspects of life. Potter argued that bioethics properly includes a heck of a lot more than that: "Medical bioethics and ecological bioethics are non-overlapping in the sense that medical bioethics is chiefly concerned with short-term views: the options open to individuals and their physicians in the attempts to prolong life by organ transplants, artificial organs, experimental chemotherapy, and all the newer developments in the field of medicine.

"In contrast, ecological bioethics clearly has a long-term view that is concerned with what we must do to preserve the ecosystem in a form that is compatible with the continued existence of the human species. These two branches of bioethics should properly overlap." (Potter, V.R. "Aldo Leopold's Land Ethic Revisited: Two Kinds of Bioethics," *Perspectives in Biology and Medicine*, Vol. 30, No. 2, Winter 1987) Truer words may never have been written.

In arguing that medical care, human health, and the biosphere are intimately intertwined, Potter cited the greatest ecological philosopher of our time, Aldo Leopold. And I believe that in his classic essay,

"The Land Ethic," Leopold offered three ideas we could use in formulating a broader ethic that reflects these deeper relationships.

First, he wrote: "An ethic, ecologically, is a limitation on freedom of action in the struggle for existence. An ethic, philosophically, is a differentiation of social from anti-social conduct. These are two definitions of one thing." (Aldo Leopold, A *Sand County Almanac*, New York City: Ballantine Books, 1966)

In other words, to harm the land is the same kind of sin as harming a human being; to protect the land is to protect humanity. The differences are not of kind, but of situation.

Second, Leopold said, there is a three-step process in the pursuit of ethical behavior, and people always seem to stop at the second step. The first step is ethics governing the individual. The second step is ethics governing relations among individuals in a society. But "there is as yet no ethic dealing with man's relation to land and to the animals and plants which grow upon it.

"Land . . . is still property. The land-relation is still strictly economic, entailing privileges but not obligations. The extension of ethics to this third element in [the] human environment is . . . an evolutionary possibility and an ecological necessity. Similarly, rather than seeking the narrowest channel and the most specialized applications, healthcare ethics should be expanding its scope.

Leopold's third observation brings all this around full circle: "All ethics so far evolved rest upon a single premise: that the individual is a member of a community of *interdependent* parts [italics mine]. The land ethic simply enlarges the boundaries of the community to include soils, waters, plants, and animals, or, collectively: the land."

Potter saw in the concept of interdependence and its inherent mutual responsibilities a means of creating "a global bioethic, an outlook that would modify the medical emphasis on individual survival and would foster peace and ecosystem preservation."

In other words, the walls we have built—between individualism and social responsibility, between self-interest and service, between the person as a medicalized ethics problem and the person as part of a biosphere, and between people as self-contained entities and people as members of an interconnected world ecology—are false and must come down.

Leopold wrote, "It is inconceivable to me that an ethical relation to land can exist without love, respect, and admiration for land: and a high regard for its value." It seems to me that an ethical relation to each other in healthcare cannot exist without our having love, respect, and admiration for our world and all its parts and peoples. Only when we have recognized this ultimate interconnectedness, and integrated it into the ethics we both preach and practice, will we have a true "bio-ethic."

But Not for Me

May 1991

O n the theoretical level, the pursuit of ethical behavior is so satisfying! One can always do the right thing. One is on the side
of the angels. One is able to construct perfect case studies, clear-cut
solutions, morally pure responses. When we discuss ethical dilemmas in theory, it's like it used to be in the movies: There is always
a happy ending.

But when it comes to applying our theoretical answers to ourselves, it's a different matter. All of a sudden, the constructs fall apart,
and what seems eminently fair on the macro-level becomes abjectly
cruel on the micro-level. All the blacks and whites dissolve into gray:

"I know that the odds of this treatment working are one in a
hundred and that it is hideously expensive, but I want to take the
chance." Or, "So what if it's a radical research experiment? This is
my child, and she should be selected for it." Or, "Of course Aunt
Grace is effectively brain-dead, but I just can't bring myself to have
the life support turned off."

Three Barriers

I think there are at least three underlying reasons for our inability
to apply the lessons and disciplines of bioethics to our own situations. And unless we understand them, most of us will continue to
risk being unable to practice what we preach.

1. Our culture is not only based on, but is in fact ruled by, individualism. In our heart of hearts, we simply prefer the individual to the group, and believe that the individual's rights hold precedence over those of the group.

This is the logical legacy of those who first came to these shores as victims of religious and class oppression. If, in your native land of England, Ireland, Germany, or wherever, your entire life was determined by the accident of your birth or by the manner in which you sought to worship, then individual rights and the chance to choose for yourself would become an obsession—as it did for those who escaped to the New World.

We still live with that obsession, which means that applying group-derived theory to our individual selves is very difficult.

2. This is also a culture of exemption. During the Reagan years, certain families that contacted the White House were able to garner a presidential plea for organ donors for children who needed transplants. Savvy parents could make direct appeals on television for donors or funds or both, and often would succeed.

Furthermore, certain people are always above the law in this society. Despite rampant malfeasance on the highest levels of government in recent years, we have not put US presidents or their children in jail. A Black rap group is tried for obscenity, and a record store owner who sells the group's music is convicted of the same crime; yet no one even blinks at Madonna, wearing red underwear, wrapping herself in the American flag, or releasing a video that many people (including the folks at MTV, who are no prudes) consider pornographic.

We apply very few standards equally to all. B.D. Colen, in his book *Hard Choices*, describes a basic healthcare conflict: In many hospitals, abortions are performed on one floor, while a few floors above, massive and sometimes hysterical efforts are made to save the lives of premature fetuses with little chance of survival. I can live with this inconsistency, because I believe the determinant must be the mother's choice, but I agree that it represents a highly differentiated application of values within one organization.

The presence of so many exemptions weakens our willingness to abide by the rules. If Leona Helmsley says that only suckers pay taxes, we who do pay them feel like fools. One can still follow one's personal morality, but one fears that it is meaningless. After all, if Exxon and Saddam Hussein foul the world's waters with oil, why should I bother to recycle?

3. Even if we are willing to apply the disciplines of bioethics to ourselves, we are much less willing to do so for those close to us. One of my favorite statistics is that although 90 percent of all health problems in adults are self-treated without resort to the healthcare system, only 25 percent of such problems in children are treated without seeking professional care. Our self-confidence fails us when the patient is not ourself, but rather a child, parent, spouse, sibling, or other loved one.

This is actually a form of altruism, in that it represents a willingness to sacrifice self and an unwillingness to sacrifice others. The fly in the ointment, of course, is that we are more than willing to sacrifice those we don't know; our altruism exists only within our own family-and-friend network.

These are old dilemmas. Alexis de Tocqueville, the French analyst who studied Americans in the 1830s, wrote in his classic *Democracy in America* about American individualism—a term he coined: "Individualism is a calm and considered feeling which disposes each citizen to isolate himself from the mass of his fellows and withdraw into the circle of family and friends; with this little society formed to his taste, he gladly leaves the greater society to look after itself. . . .

"Such folk owe no man anything and hardly expect anything from anybody. They form the habit of thinking of themselves in isolation and imagine that their whole destiny is in their own hands. Thus not only does democracy make men forget their ancestors, but also clouds their view of their descendants and isolates them from their contemporaries. Each man is forever thrown back on himself alone, and there is danger that he may be shut up in the solitude of his own heart."

Wrenching Self-Examination

In such a society, can we ever hope to make tough bioethical rules stick? Can we really ration care, pull the plug, change values, think communally, and accept the dominance of social theories in our personal lives?

I hope so. I think we must, or we might as well junk our efforts to develop a socioethical underpinning for healthcare, and go fishing instead. But it is incredibly difficult to subject ourselves and those we love to such discipline; it requires wrenching self-examination. As part of that self-scrutiny, I have the following thoughts on combating the three barriers I just described.

First, in terms of individualism, the fact remains that no individual life in this (or any other) society makes any sense except as a function of the larger group. Indeed, an individual who scorns the bonds of society is generally dubbed a sociopath.

And a society does not exist as a theory; it consists of the interrelationships of those who people it. If we are unwilling to be bound by its rules, then street traffic becomes violent chaos, laws become unenforceable, environmental responsibility becomes meaningless, and the law of the jungle prevails.

In forming a society in the first place, our species agreed to the most basic of tradeoffs: I will accept the discipline of the group, if the group will offer me protection. So if the group requires a certain sacrifice or a certain behavior, we must offer it; otherwise no one is safe. By being responsible members of a group society, we protect our individualism.

As for exemptions: Given that we resent those who benefit by being exempted from the rules, we simply need to be much tougher about who is exempted, and why. We need to adjust a situation in which wealthy felons serve far less prison time (if any at all) than poor ones.

Dave Barry of the *Miami Herald* recently joked that Michael Milken, the junk-bond trader who was convicted of fraud, came up with the $600 million he was assessed in fines by selling his watch. Oliver North has made far more money on the speaking circuit than he paid in fines for breaking the law. Imelda Marcos (had she been convicted) could have paid her penalties out of petty cash. People should not be able to buy their way off the hook so easily.

If we are not supposed to seek unjustifiable exemption for ourselves, we cannot tolerate it for others. In fact, we may tolerate it being granted to others as a means of securing an escape for ourselves, should we need it. But every exemption, every end-run, every flouting of the law—be it a governmental law or a moral law—weakens that law and allows more exemptions. In the end, the law—as we learned so clearly during the era of Prohibition—becomes toothless. And when exemption is the rule, then random justice (or injustice) is the order of the day.

And what do we do when the person to whom the bioethical decision should apply is someone close to us but not ourselves? We need to question frankly whether our hesitance to apply appropriate principles and decisions to that person is based in a desire to protect them, or in a wish to protect ourselves.

I have become convinced that much of the time, we are unwilling to terminate treatment or refuse a dubious course of care or challenge a decision because of our own selfishness, not because of a need to protect someone else.

Let's face it: If a cesarean section is inappropriate for me under given conditions, it is equally inappropriate for my sister or my daughter under those conditions. If I am terrified of being lashed to some form of life-prolonging technology, I should be equally terrified that someone I love will be subjected to the same imprisonment.

There are two motivations at work here. One is our basic individualistic desire not to tell anyone else what to do, which is often misdirected. The other, more powerful issue is that we fear accountability; we do not want to be responsible for the consequences of our decisions regarding someone else. All I can say to this is that we should not undervalue ourselves, nor should we overvalue others, when it comes to such decisions.

If Karen Ann Quinlan's parents and Nancy Cruzan's parents and Paul Brophy's family could stand up and say to the world, "This is enough—stop it!," certainly the rest of us can do the same.

The baseline in all ethical decisions is accountability, whether in the global arena of policy, the macro-arena of resource allocation within the hospital, or the micro-arena of me or a member of my family. If the decision would be right for me, it's right for those I love; if it is wrong for me, it is wrong for them.

If we are willing to look it in the face, the difficulty in applying ethical principles to ourselves is not a soul-crushing dilemma. It is a matter of understanding that we all live as part of a larger group to which we must have some loyalty. It is a matter of expecting and seeking to ensure that the rules are applied equally to all unless there is a *very* good reason for an exception. And it is a matter of having the courage to take responsibility for our own decisions and to accept their consequences. As far as I'm concerned, all that is simply part of being a grownup.

Ethics and the Quality of Care

July 1991

There is a great deal of interest these days in new approaches to healthcare quality assurance: "continuous quality improvement" (CQI), "total quality management" (TQM), and the like. These are very appealing concepts, rooted in the idea that the pursuit of quality should be a positive striving for betterment rather than a negative hunt for bad apples.

In addition, these new approaches seek to improve quality prospectively, rather than retrospectively. And they encourage the involvement of everyone in the organization, rather than confining quality activities to the quality assurance committee, which no one ever wants to serve on, anyway.

I welcome these approaches, with some reservations. One is that these ideas, like many elements in the new wave of objective measurement of quality, are being oversold; they are not a magic bullet. They are providing a fertile field of endeavor for consultants, but they will not solve all our problems.

Even more important, as Professor Leon Wyszewianski of the University of Michigan has pointed out, CQI and TQM can easily become an elaborate form of "cheerleading" that puts more pressure on housekeepers and food service staff than on the clinical staff, and expresses more concern over whether the food is hot than over repeated readmissions for infection.

Nevertheless, the growing interest in these new ways of seeking to improve quality provides me with an excuse to discuss the ethical dimensions of quality assurance in healthcare.

Provider Ambivalence

On the surface, quality assurance as an ethical imperative should not be a real tough sell. Seeking to provide the very best care possible, and attempting to improve that high level of care, is obviously the only moral choice healthcare providers have. After all, how could one possibly defend the conscious provision of substandard care?

Yet many providers do not see quality assurance as an ethics issue. Instead, one hears about avoiding malpractice litigation, the need to comply with Joint Commission on Accreditation of Healthcare Organizations standards, or the drive to remain competitive. Behind the words is a kind of foot-dragging mentality reflecting a widespread attitude that quality assurance is a nuisance, not an opportunity or a moral responsibility. Why is that?

There are several reasons that we have not linked quality and ethics. For one thing, the focus of public attention on the quality of care is quite recent. It was born, in many ways, with Medicare prospective payment. Faced with shorter lengths of stay and alleged restrictions on funding (which was hardly the case in 1983 and 1984, when most hospitals made out like bandits under prospective payment systems), hospitals and physicians raised the cry of quality in order to prevent restrictions from being imposed on them. This was in keeping with the "more is better" standard of healthcare quality, which had been the traditional benchmark.

What happened, of course, is that the quality of care went public, aided no end by the scandals over the deaths of Andy Warhol and other patients. We are only now adjusting to the movement of quality assurance out of the dusty medical records review office and onto the front page of the *Los Angeles Times*. And we are not at all sure we like our quality activities and problems being splashed all over the papers.

Furthermore, frankly, many providers raised the spectre of compromised quality, not because they were all that worried about the vulnerability of patients but rather as a means of keeping the money flowing. They predicted dire results if the flow of funds was constrained. (In the United Kingdom, this is called "shroud waving.") So in some cases, the sudden concern about quality was probably not entirely sincere.

A Tender Trap

In trying to use quality to protect financing, providers fell into the same trap in which many payers have fallen: confusing quality with cost. The two sides are lined up along opposing edges of a trench. The providers are still saying that more is better, and quality is best protected by spending more money; the payers are saying that less is better, and that quality is best protected by limiting spending. Too often it's the patient who falls into the trench between them.

The entry of payers into the fray provided another reason for providers to be ambivalent about quality assurance: It signaled the intrusion of powerful outside interests into what healthcare thought was its own business. Traditionally, quality was what we said it was: Take our word for it, we're doing a great job. Providers controlled quality assessment and cloaked it in secrecy, draping it with highly technical language and clinical concepts that few of the rest of us could understand even if we wanted to.

Healthcare was used to being on the honor system where quality was concerned: No one else could understand, and no one else should be allowed to participate. It was our turf. We demanded, and received, the cloak of confidentiality. Only physicians were allowed to examine and discipline physicians. We even resented and derided the efforts of the Joint Commission, a provider-based organization.

And providers thought they were doing a good job under the honor system. Unfortunately, that did not prove to be the case, and word started leaking out. There was "Dr. X," injecting helpless patients with curare in an East Coast hospital, whose license wasn't even lifted. There was the notorious Dr. Burt in a midwestern hospital, who for years butchered the genitals of women while they were under anesthesia—in full view of doubting physicians who nevertheless did not intervene.

There were murderous nurses and anesthesiologists who raped patients while they were unconscious and entire hospitals with mortality rates so high that even the most stubborn data-hater would have reason to question the quality of their services. The Public Citizen Health Research Group started publishing cesarean rates for individual hospitals, some of them exceeding 50 percent.

And healthcare did little or nothing. If a physician was found incompetent, the usual procedure was to write glowing letters of recommendation and send him or her to the next hospital along the line. Really bad eggs would be encouraged to set up practice in another state. More often, however, other physicians would cover for the substandard work of colleagues, and woe betide the nurse or technician who tried to call attention to the problem. It wasn't an honor system; it was a buddy system.

And it failed, because, in the words of former New York State health commissioner David Axelrod, MD, "Doctors forgot the difference between what they owe to other professionals and what they owe to their profession." And what we got was the National Practitioner Data Bank, erosion of confidentiality, and massive outside intervention in quality assurance. When honor systems fail, you get regulations and laws in their stead.

Quality as Morality

So yes, there are many reasons for health care professionals to think of quality assurance as a millstone around their necks. It *is* a heavy responsibility; it *should* be taken seriously. However, it's not a burden so much as it is a chance to be better and to do better, to discharge honorably the duty to protect patients, and to preserve the privilege of being viewed as a special sector of society.

Nevertheless, as you launch organization-wide quality assurance programs, and cooperative data-sharing programs with other institutions in your state or network or system, and deploy more objective, scientifically based methods of evaluating the quality of care, you may hear some grumping in the back pew.

Let me suggest a few thoughts you can shoot back:

Protecting patients is the healthcare professional's highest calling. Providers have, first and foremost, two ethical responsibilities. One is to ensure that all people, regardless of income or race or diagnosis, have access to necessary healthcare on a timely basis (we haven't done too well with that one, either, but that's another column). The other is to ensure that patients receive the best possible care.

Patients have a right to expect that they will be treated competently and humanely, that their dignity will be honored, and their physical and emotional health safeguarded. We owe that to them and to the society that invests its trust in us. These are our primary ethical responsibilities, not protecting professional standing, nor making scientific breakthroughs, nor advancing the use of new technologies. Protect patients first.

We are all responsible for everyone's patients. My two major concerns about payer-driven quality assurance are that first, if you're paying for it, you shouldn't also be deciding if it should be done, because the conflict of interest is too great. Second, payers only care about the quality of services provided to the people they're paying for; to hell with everyone else.

In a system like that, who speaks for the uninsured poor? Who evaluates the quality of their care?

Beyond that, the fact is that we are all responsible for all patients, whether we treat them or not. If we know there is a bad doctor, a substandard hospital, a questionable program, or a dangerous ambulance out there, it is our responsibility to protect patients who might fall victim to them. That is what was so heinous about our long-standing practice of simply sending dangerous doctors to the hospital next door. How can we claim that our patients are more valuable than their patients?

It is not enough to ensure the quality of care of patients within our own personal purview. We need to ensure the quality of care of all patients—and of those who should be patients but are denied access.

Most patients are not with us voluntarily. Despite all the talk about healthcare being an "industry" and health services being just another commodity like sneakers, there is one teeny difference: Most of our customers are not here by choice, and most of the purchases they make are involuntary. They are also often scared out of their minds, feverish, bleeding, perhaps even dying. All told, if given the choice, most patients would rather be in Philadelphia. Given their lack of options, to betray them with poor care is a moral offense far more serious than selling them the wrong kind of running shoe. It's all well and good to say *"caveat emptor"* to an informed, healthy consumer; it's another thing to say it to someone who was just run over by a dump truck.

Traditional yardsticks remain important. When a fad sweeps through healthcare quality assurance—regardless of its usefulness—there is always a danger that managers will turn away from the complexities and frustrations of clinical quality assurance to easier approaches, like using patient satisfaction surveys (despite the fact that most patients don't know if they needed the operation or not), redecorating the birthing suite, or yelling at the housekeeping staff.

The fact is that the most dangerous things in a hospital or nursing home are not the food (not usually, anyway) but rather clinical treatments and procedures, post-treatment care, and the hygiene of the environment. Even with all the good that CQI and TQM have to offer, remember that we must start with ruthless assurance of good clinical quality and hygiene, and that the three yardsticks defined by Avedis Donabedian decades ago—structure, process, and outcome— are still the standard.

It isn't just how well you do it, it's whether you should do it. True quality assurance goes beyond evaluating the quality of the action taken to determining whether it should be taken. With many procedures—cesarean, coronary artery bypass grafts, carotid endart-erectomy, a fifth liver transplant in the same child—there is compelling evidence of overuse.

An ethical commitment to quality assurance also means a com-mitment to acting only when necessary. As Eugenia Hamilton of the Dartmouth-Hitchcock Medical Center has said, "There is no point in doing something well if you shouldn't be doing it in the first place."

This also means we must demonstrate the results of what we choose to do—the outcomes-based approach. If the outcome is poor, we must rethink what we are doing immediately. That can make for problems, as there are some real black holes in healthcare— chemical dependency programs, certain mental health services, eating disorders clinics, *in vitro* fertilization—for which outcomes information is discouraging. Yet these programs are proliferating like wildfire.

If we mean what we say about quality assurance, we have to take on all these challenges: how well we do what we do, whether we should do it at all, what the results are, and how many of us should be doing it. That will be anything but easy. But if we are willing to make this kind of commitment, we will accomplish three things: We will be protecting our patients to the very best of our ability. We will move quality assurance beyond window-dressing to a rock-solid, scientific basis. And we will preserve the honor of the healthcare system. It certainly seems worth the effort.

. . . .

What Happens Because of How We Choose

The Case of Children

September 1991

Unfortunately, since this column was written, the plight of low-income children (and many other children) has gotten worse. Our urban immunization rate is 50%; in rural areas, it is 60%. For minority children, it is lower than even those pitiful figures. Fordham University reported in 1995 that the rate of child abuse in the United States had hit a new high, as had the number of children living in poverty. More than 10 million children have no health insurance. Children have died of measles and chicken pox in California and elsewhere. The debate may rage about saddling tomorrow's children with the national debt, but too many of today's children won't be alive to hear it.

In keeping with my belief that most issues in ethics boil down to the making of choices (hence the name of this column), this is a story about the options we have and why we pick the ones we do. This tale fits playwright Arthur Miller's definition of tragedy: failure in the presence of the possibility of success.

In the United States in 1990, in this richest of all nations, with what claims to be the finest of all healthcare systems, there were 26,500 reported cases of measles. (The actual total, because of under-reporting, may have been twice that.) At least 68 children under the age of 19 died of this disease, which we have known how to prevent, through immunization, for decades.

This is not only tragic but mysterious. We are spending billions of dollars to find ways to prevent other diseases, such as cancer and AIDS, and billions more to treat other conditions that afflict children, such as organ failures that require expensive and often dicey transplants. We are constantly complaining about the cost of last-minute care. Yet immunization—inexpensive, easy, and the most effective single tool in the entire healthcare armamentarium—is declining in terms of the number of children reached.

The American Academy of Pediatrics estimates that 40 percent of children under age five are not immunized against measles; consensus estimates are that 25 percent of our children are not properly immunized against childhood diseases. It's hard to know, exactly, because the federal government withdrew funding for collection of immunization data in 1985, making it very difficult for states and localities to fill the gap and thus essentially making national data unavailable. Another case of hiding the evidence, if you ask me.

How has this happened? It was the perfectly logical result of a series of choices made by society in general and the healthcare system in particular, and it provides a valuable, if awful, lesson in how hidden agendas can harm and kill. Here are the options we had, and the choices we made.

Us Versus Them

Many of the children who contract measles, and die from it, are nonwhite. Of three major outbreaks last year, one occurred among Samoan children in the Los Angeles area, one occurred among Southeast Asian children in the Central Valley of California, and a third occurred among black children in Philadelphia. All three communities were low-income to boot. When I asked a California official about the Central Valley outbreak, he responded casually, "Oh, the children who died were Southeast Asian, and their parents don't bring them in for immunization."

Gee, I hate to tell the man his business, but I thought public health was supposed to be outward-looking and community-oriented in its strategies. Should the health department just sit around and watch an epidemic develop because the victims—many of them the children of immigrants—aren't coming in to be immunized? Or should public health people go to where the need is? Immunization is not common in many Third World nations; maybe families don't know it's available. And should we, as a nation, so underfund public health departments that they may have no choice but to sit and watch?

I hardly think it's acceptable to allow people to emigrate from a situation of no access to healthcare in their own countries to a similar situation here in the Land of Opportunity. And I doubt that an epidemic among suburban white kids would be similarly ignored.

Because ours is a largely white, middle-class healthcare system, reflecting a largely white society, an epidemic among those who are different, who are "the other," to use writer Toni Morrison's phrase, is not "our" crisis. It was a mistake we made when AIDS first appeared among gay men. It is a mistake we are making again.

Now or Later

Our healthcare system, egged on by society and the news media, has found its glory in the last-minute save, the skin-of-the-teeth intervention, the pulling back of the patient from the grave. It's healthcare's answer to the home run in the bottom of the ninth inning, what Ron Anderson, MD, director of Parkland Memorial Hospital in Dallas, calls "resurrection medicine." As a result, the entire system is pitched to rushing in at the last minute.

That does not put early-intervention care in a position of high prestige, to put it mildly. Thus prevention and early diagnosis and treatment remain a professional backwater, even as payers and government frantically try to contain costs and improve health status.

The situation is exacerbated by what Albert Jonsen of the University of Washington refers to as "the rule of rescue"—our basic need to throw the life preserver to the individual most in danger of drowning, even if others have a greater chance of survival.

In the face of these deeply embedded priorities, immunization could not be expected to fare well in the absence of a systemwide ethical commitment to protect our children. That commitment has not been forthcoming.

Prevention Versus Cure

This is a companion choice to the previous one. Preventive medicine suffers from the same problem as public health medicine: Success is measured in the absence of problems. In a cure-oriented system, we count our triumphs in terms of cancers in remission, hearts healed, bones set, ulcers abated. We don't know how to count epidemics that did not take place, food poisoning that did not occur, cholera that did not affect the water supply.

As a result, the healthcare system has been able to grab most of the resources for curative care, while prevention has languished. This is reflected in the absurdity of a health insurance system in which 55 percent of private insurers do not cover immunization (more of them cover transplants than measles shots). Medicare only decided to cover mammography last year—and that was the result of massive public pressure. Until we include protection of little kids in our litany of glamorous forms of care, preventive services will remain in the back of the healthcare bus.

Public Versus Private

Ours is a largely private healthcare system, which has its advantages and its drawbacks; but it does mean that the private usually takes precedence over the public. And immunization, traditionally, has been disproportionately publicly funded and conducted by public providers—public health workers, community health centers, public hospitals, and others. It is just not a type of care in which the private sector has shown all that much interest.

Indeed, recent American Academy of Pediatrics research indicates that referrals of children in need of immunization to public clinics by private providers has risen in recent years. But the public sector is overloaded. Community health centers report that they are chronically short of vaccines: 71 percent report recent shortages of vaccines for measles, mumps, rubella, and pertussis. This is just one more example of what happens when a societal and healthcare system responsibility is abandoned to an underfunded, overworked public sector.

Adults Versus Children

There are few areas of public policy in which there is more variance between what we say we believe, and what we actually do, than the health of children. We all profess to a desire to protect the next generation; indeed, the ongoing battle over abortion has been cast in terms of fetal and child rights. In the transplant derby, children are far more likely to garner donated funds and organs than are adults. As Charlie Fiske, father of Jamie Fiske, the first heavily publicized pediatric liver recipient, said, "Dogs and kids get all the attention."

In terms of public sentiment, we are still captured by the tenet of major religions that children are born innocent and thus are more worthy of our protection and attention than are adults. We have laws governing child labor and banning child abuse and neglect and child pornography.

Too bad we don't find society's neglect and abandonment of its children's health obscene; maybe we could outlaw it. As it is, 12 million children live in poverty, 11 million lack healthcare coverage, and 6 million go to bed hungry every night here in this child-loving nation.

I do not believe that the measles epidemic would have been allowed to get this far among adults. Why, then, did we abandon children to it? Because what the director of a community mental health center in Alabama once said of his clients is equally true of children: "There's not a vote in a carload." And when it comes to holes yawning open in our supposed safety nets, it is the littlest bodies that fall through first.

Individual Versus Collective Action

Many health problems can be addressed individually: I cut my hand, I get it stitched. Others, like epidemics among underserved populations, must be addressed collectively, by a wide range of entities—physicians, hospitals, social service agencies, schools, governments, news media, and third-party payers. Fighting measles and the other threats lurking out there—polio and tuberculosis among them—means a broad-based, collective form of healthcare that is not as attractive as the individual, personalized kind of care.

Furthermore, it means taking other people's problems on as our own. I have heard, repeatedly, that the lack of childhood immunization is the parents' fault. Great. Let's not blame it on the systemic failure that underlies it; let's individualize the problem and pin it on parents who may or may not "know better."

I have a better idea. Why don't we admit that we, as a society and as a healthcare system, made a series of choices—and made them very lightly at that? And now children are paying the price of those choices. Why don't we reconsider, and recast, those choices, rather than seeking to blame this disaster on some specific villain who is not us? We can't individualize everything in healthcare, try as we might. Some problems we must address together—all of us.

That was our most perverse choice. Neilson Buchanan, chief executive officer of El Camino Hospital in Mountain View, California, has spoken eloquently about the epidemic and how it happened: "Our common sense and our sense of community failed at the same time." It is time we revived both.

There are signs of hope. President Bush and Secretary Sullivan recently made heavily publicized announcements about increasing immunization rates. (However, they appear unwilling or unable to back up those promises with any kind of extra funding.) The Junior Leagues of Ohio, in partnership with the Children's Defense Fund and several hospitals, have inaugurated a year-long campaign to immunize every child in the state. All hospitals in New York City, public and private, are cooperating in the "Assignment Good Health" program, which seeks to provide appropriate preventive services, including immunization, to every child entering the school system. And both the American Academy of Pediatrics and the Children's Defense Fund have been increasingly visible in their passionate advocacy for these littlest and most powerless of patients.

But we are a long way from accepting the consequences of our choices as a society, let alone making better decisions in the future. Until we understand what happens as a result of the options we select, we will still, unintentionally, be causing death, disability, and suffering. We will remain guilty of what Raul Alfonsin, the first civilian president of Argentina after the military dictatorship fell in 1983, said of his own nation: "When a country that signified life for the millions who came here kills its own children, then we have touched rock bottom."

Rationing Healthcare

Crisis and Courage

November 1991

Healthcare and health policy are in crisis. It is said there is not enough money to go around (at least under current resource allocation arrangements). Health status indicators are declining. Counties are at war with states, and states with the federal government, over who should pay for the Medicaid and uninsured populations.

Healthcare system reform inspires much debate but little action in Congress, and is a nonevent at the White House. Meanwhile, Rome burns. And everyone is talking about the need to ration care—only to someone else, of course. But everyone agrees on the need to do it.

So we engage in polite discussions about how to deny what to whom in an ethical manner. I've participated in my share of such discussions, and I've asked my share of the standard rationing questions. But recently, after teaching a course on the subject at Boston University, I was reminded of a line from Arthur Penn's film, *Night Moves*. At one point, a detective is vainly trying to get some information from a mysterious woman. He begs and wheedles and pleads, but she insists on responding to him with obscurities that make no sense. Finally, he explodes, "Why can't you give me a straight answer?" She says, "Because you're asking the wrong questions."

I have come to believe that, in terms of the crisis in healthcare policy and rationing, we are asking the wrong questions. After all, there are ways to ration healthcare on both the micro and macro levels that are more or less damaging, more or less hypocritical, more or less democratic, and more or less acceptable in the eyes of God and humanity. Which methods are used is decided by politics, whether it's an election year, how the press sees the situation, and a hundred other arbitrary factors. In reducing healthcare to a monetarized, sterile set of budget items, one does the best one can.

But those choices are made in the context of broader questions. And those questions are even less comfortable than whether Oregon should refuse to fund treatment of the damaged Achilles tendons or lymphomas or AIDS of some of its most vulnerable residents. Indeed, now that the waiver process is under way in Oregon, we will undoubtedly be treated to a slew of dainty ethics articles in all the correct journals, arguing whether providers have the moral right to refuse to provide these services to destitute patients. I fear we will have to suffer through these appeals to God and Hippocrates for months. In this time of crisis, hypocrisy is triumphing over human decency.

But that debate, too, will in all probability avoid the basic questions underlying it. So let me ask three of those questions. They concern the context within which we ration and whether what we choose is acceptable—defining "acceptable" as what we can do while still holding our heads reasonably high.

Whose Interest Are We Serving?

I believe that the rationing debate is rooted, not in issues of human service or public policy, but rather in political convenience. We pull all the really scary cards out of the deck before we start dealing. Before we begin work on the budget, before we start deciding who will be denied, we have already made all the important choices.

We will not do anything that will jeopardize our jobs. We will not do anything that will lose us too many votes in the next election. We will not do anything to embarrass (a) the governor, (b) the legislature, (c) the Speaker or Majority Leader, (d) the party. We will not jeopardize campaign funding. We will not mention income taxes. We will not take on anyone too powerful. We will not take on the privately insured or their insurance carriers.

So it can never come down to reallocating the embarrassment of riches in healthcare. We prattle about not being able to afford to treat leg injuries in children while sitting in the middle of a $750 billion pig-out! Instead, it always comes down to cutting Medicaid, general assistance health funds, public hospital funds, public health nursing, immunization. It comes down to who and what cannot fight back.

When this happens, policy is simply reflecting society—this enclave society, this us-and-them world, where we take pride in having caused the deaths of some 200,000 people in Iraq because they were not Americans. This cowering society has told its public servants that the poor, the vulnerable, the crazy, the homeless, the helpless are not our problem; they are no part of us. Besides, they deserve what happens to them.

We will not pay for liver transplants for people with alcoholic cirrhosis, but we will pay for liver transplants for people with liver cancer—even though the chance of survival is the same for both groups. We are increasingly resistant to public funding of AIDS care, as the patient profile becomes that of a much less powerful population than earlier patients. These are not clinical decisions; these are social decisions, based on the corrupting values of a society that is playing Pontius Pilate with parts of itself.

One of my rules of rationing is that someone always gets hurt. I accept that. If there is not a sufficient amount of something people need (what they *want* is a different issue), then someone is going to get hurt. But it is unlikely to be white, middle-class me who gets hurt. It is always the same people. And the reason they get hurt is that they are far more dependent on government, while being far less able to influence it, than the rest of us.

Perhaps we should remember that the reason they are the province of government is that there is no one else to speak for and protect them. And if government abandons them, then they are truly, and tragically, alone. These most vulnerable people, far from serving as targets, should be the special concern of society. They should be the focus, not of our neglect, but of our attention.

But this does not happen; instead, we disdain them, citing their alleged lack of moral fortitude, their unemployment, their lack of hygiene or sanity, their lack of stick-to-it-iveness. And when society does this, at a moment of crisis, what is government's response? To bow to the will of the people and join the mob.

The resource we are lacking in the rationing debate is not money; it is political courage. It is leadership. It is the once-glorious tradition in this country of people who sought to serve in the public sector because of a desire for change, not a desire to preserve a dysfunctional status quo—of people who wanted to challenge whether this was how things had to be.

Thank God for those health policymakers who still believe that first, you lead; first, you have vision; first, you insist on what is right. Then you try to save your job. And thank God for the electorates who came through for them because they came through for humanity.

For it is in the darkest of budgetary times, when it is so easy to say there is no money for unpopular people or programs, that people of courage must draw the line and say: "This will not do. If there must be more suffering, then let us all do a little of it. I will not continue to kick children, even if that is what you want me to do."

What Are the Long-Term Consequences of Our Actions?

In this short-term world, where long-range planning ends at the next fiscal year, we do not consider the long-term effects of what we do. What happens as a result are AIDS and measles epidemics, a collapsing rural health system, inner-city healthcare deserts, a teetering public health system, and 35 million people without coverage. Yet when we finally notice these consequences, our response, more often than not, is a frenzied attempt to hide the evidence.

The late Graham Greene wrote *The Quiet American,* a book about the beginnings of the American experience in Vietnam. In it, the narrator describes a supremely naive American operative, who, in pursuing his wildly skewed vision of American interests, provokes a group of radicals to engage in an act of terrorism that kills and maims a large number of people. The narrator, enraged at the carnage, starts to explain to the American what he has done. But then he says to himself, "What's the good? He'll always be innocent; you can't blame the innocent. They are always guiltless. All you can do is control them or eliminate them. Innocence is a kind of insanity."

That destructive innocence underlies our inability to understand the consequences of our decisions. Someone always gets hurt by rationing, but the worst hurts may not be the immediate results. The long-term results may be far more harmful. In our innocence, we do not understand that the real threat involved in rationing care too tightly is the inevitable downward spiral that results.

We decide to stop funding a few services under Medicaid, and within a few years we are funding virtually none. We decide that a 95 percent immunization rate is sufficient, and soon it is 50 percent. We figure that it is easier to build a few shelters than to regulate the real estate market, and soon there are tens of thousands of homeless families. These are the results of policy decisions made years or decades ago.

We need backstops. We must incorporate long-term thinking into our rationing decisions, so that the necessary safeguards can be built in. We need to be able to stop the downward spiral. Otherwise the insanity of our innocence will lead us to a gallows where we may all hang, in time.

On Whose Hands Should the Blood Be?

This has to do with the civic agony of Milwaukee, and with a person of political courage, John O. Norquist, the mayor of that tortured city. He recently conceded that if mass murderer Jeffrey

Dahmer had been Black, he would have been stopped earlier. I would add that if Jeffrey Dahmer's victims had been white, rather than Black and Laotian, he also would have been stopped earlier.

But, as the *Chicago Tribune* pointed out, most of the people who were killed lived at the fringes. They rode buses to another city to engage in a secret lifestyle. They were presumed by police in several cities to be the kind of people who could be expected to disappear. They were not connected.

In *The Care of Strangers*, his brilliant history of American hospitals, Charles Rosenberg points out that the people who ended up in the almshouses were not connected in society; they did not have a web of human relationships around them. In that case, government afforded them protection, in the form of the early public hospitals. In Milwaukee, government let them go quietly and unnoticed to their deaths.

Now blood lust is rising: There is a massive push to find a way to execute Jeffrey Dahmer. Even in Wisconsin, which has not had the death penalty for 140 years, an effort is under way to reinstate it. Why? Revenge, of course. Most litigation, as attorney Eric Springer says, is an act of vengeance. And capital punishment is the ultimate vengeance of society.

But revenge is really a secondary reason. The main motivation for our wanting to kill Dahmer is our own sense of guilt: the guilt of a police department, a neighborhood, a city, a state, a nation, and a society that allowed or even enabled an obscene string of social failures and moral abandonments that led, in the end, to mass murder.

The pattern is easily seen: cover-ups by families, friends, and others who looked the other way when strange behavior occurred. A probation officer who was excused from visiting the apartment because it was in a "bad neighborhood." Homophobic police. A homophobic society that encouraged the secret lifestyles that disconnected the victims from those who would notice they were gone. Racism. Cynicism. The unfashionability of getting involved. The dismissal of those few who did want to get involved.

Just as cowardice killed Kitty Genovese in New York City a generation ago, these failings killed those young men. And we all did it. Maybe someone should stop us before we kill again, but it is easier to turn the mirror to the wall and seek to execute the representative of our collective failure.

Must care be denied? Must people suffer? Must children die? Perhaps that is how it must be for now, until we recover our sense of humanity. But if those who serve as representatives of the people are brought to this pass, I hope they will not continue to be so polite about doing our bidding. They should not, to use Dylan Thomas' words, "go gentle into that good night." They should read the rest of us in on the act. They should not excuse us by saying that it won't hurt, or people will not suffer, or it's okay—just this once. Pontius Pilate, after all, is not remembered as a paragon of good government.

Our policymakers should turn around to the rest of us and say: "This is your work, too. This is the tradeoff your votes and preferences and pollsters have dictated. This is partially your fault. Some of this blood is on your hands. If you can live with that, fine; I will do your will for as long as I can stomach it. But if you do not want to live with it, then for God's sake, let us, together, find another way."

I often quote philosopher Philip Hallie, who studies the tangled morality of the Nazi era. He served in World War II and is haunted by acts he committed while in the military. Yet he has also said he believes that pacifism, even if it was the more morally attractive course, would not have stopped Hitler. He says it took decent men like himself becoming killers to stop Hitler. That was what Joseph Goebbels said—that to stop the Nazis, the enemy would have to become like them.

But, Hallie says, altruistic motivation does not excuse us when we violate moral law. Even if it is necessary to stop a greater evil, killing extracts a price from those who commit it. Even in time of war, when law, custom, and society indemnify the killer, morality does not. And so, Hallie says, the killer pays a price. In Hallie's case, he will hear artillery ringing in his ears for the rest of his life. In my case, for my partial responsibility—however indirect—for what happened in Milwaukee, it will be a different price. It is different in each case.

The important thing is that a price must be paid for causing hurt, and it must be paid by all of us. Thus it does not serve us well if our political leaders continue to accept the blame for what we have all done. If we bring them to account, so must they bring us to account. If we ask them to do the difficult or the unspeakable, they must remind us that they do it on our behalf. If there must be blood, it must be on all our hands.

Without that essential and terrible knowledge, times of crisis will continue to be used as an excuse for doing the inexcusable with impunity. And without that essential and terrible knowledge, there is no such thing as democracy.

. . . .

This article is based on a presentation made to the National Academy for State Health Policy annual conference in Denver on August 5, 1991.

The Ethics of Empires

March 1992

The move to integrated healthcare organizations that provide a comprehensive range of services to patients in a community or region is long overdue. Indeed, as one watches the march of organizations like the Kaiser Foundation Health Plan through the patient care markets of California and elsewhere, one is tempted to ask what took the rest of healthcare so long in terms of emulating and adapting that model.

Whenever there is an issue of new structures, new organizations, and new missions, however, there is also an issue of how ethics problems and discussions will be handled. And in the rush to formulate new forms of capitation, financing, and employer contracting, the need for new ethics structures tends to get lost in the shuffle. This is not surprising.

Despite great progress in the establishment of ethics committees, policies on the use of cardiopulmonary resuscitation, and procedures for implementing the Patient Self-Determination Act, I don't think anyone working in biomedical ethics would claim that every healthcare organization has licked the problem of how to deal with ethics consultations. Even if organizational structures are in place, compliance on the part of staff members remains spotty, in many cases.

What Is Needed?

How should ethics education, discussion, and consultation be handled in these new healthcare organizations—especially those that are the result of combining existing organizations, and/or those that now offer a variety of services, such as acute inpatient care, outpatient services, longterm care, meals and social services for the elderly, and outreach?

Begin with what's there. What ethics structures are already in place? Does each of the participating hospitals (if there is more than one involved in the new organization) have an ethics advisory committee? That might well be the case. Does the longterm care component have an ethics committee? Probably not. If there are group practices involved, they are unlikely to have ethics committees of their own, although members of the practice may well serve on hospital committees. Outpatient, outreach, and sociomedical services probably don't have their own ethics structures (with the exception of home healthcare agencies, some of which have them or else can avail themselves of ethics advisory committees at their parent organizations).

Once an inventory of existing ethics structures has been conducted (and in some organizations, unfortunately, that won't take long), it helps to find out how well they have been working. Probably the best way to accomplish this without ruffling feathers is to ask a bioethicist from another organization or an ethics consultant to conduct an evaluation of the effectiveness of the various committees or other entities that have provided ethics counseling.

This evaluation process is best initiated, in my opinion, at the board level of the integrated organization. If a request for review of ethics activity comes from lower down in the organization, the review may well become embroiled in the inevitable turf battles that accompany the merger or acquisition of multiple healthcare entities. Therefore, evaluative activity should be instigated by the overall board and should be conducted with extreme caution and sensitivity. There is probably enough nervousness within the organization without adding concerns about whether the ethics committee or consulting service is going to be dismantled.

Once the evaluation has been conducted and its findings digested, three other steps are necessary:

1. Fix what's wrong. This is simply a matter of learning from the evaluation and from the experience of those who have been working with extant ethics entities, whether as members or as those who have sought consultation or education. This should be done periodically by all ethics consultation and education entities. However, as with everything else, self-evaluation is hard and outside evaluation is resented, so very often ethics committees can go on their merry way for years without being scrutinized very closely. They are, after all, doing God's work, so even those who feel that work could be done better are loath to intervene.

The formation of a new organization thus provides an outstanding opportunity for a little soul-searching and self-examination— even on the part of committees who think they are doing a good job. And again, outside help from sister organizations, independent ethics consultants from academia, or elsewhere can make the process a little less prickly.

2. Institute what's missing. This is really just a process of recognizing that many new healthcare organizations do not offer consistent access to ethics consultation and discussion. Most hospitals have ethics committees; most integrated healthcare organizations do not. Thus the hospital ethics committee (or committees) may be stretched to handle consultations in the realm of home healthcare, outpatient services, group practice management, or even Meals on Wheels.

I do not believe this is the best way to go, for three reasons. First, particularly if more than one ethics committee already existed in what are now the parts of a new organization, turf battles are almost inevitable. If, say, a Catholic hospital merges with a Seventh-Day Adventist hospital (which is unlikely, but a Jewish hospital merged with an Episcopal facility a few years ago in New York City), the new organization could inherit two ethics committees, each of which had been the primary source of hospital ethics consultation, and each of which is operating on the basis of distinct values. Which one will dominate the new organization? Probably the best answer is neither; rather than allowing them to duke it out, form a new one that includes members of previous committees who are capable of collaboration.

Second, even if there is only one hospital involved in the formation of the new organization, those staff members and employees who were working in nonhospital, non-inpatient settings are not necessarily going to be thrilled with seeking guidance from a committee whose only previous experience was with acute inpatient care. Nursing homes, home healthcare, outpatient clinics, and other structures all deal with different ethics issues.

Furthermore, their populations are often very different from the patient mix in a general hospital. In many hospitals, elderly patients are in the minority; in nursing homes, they constitute almost the entire caseload—and most of them are the same gender, to boot. A home healthcare worker is toiling in a very different environment from that of the surgical suite—and very often must make independent decisions away from the parent organization.

Also, acute-care hospitals—especially teaching hospitals—have been the "stars" of the healthcare system, garnering most of the prestige, power, and money. People who have been working in nonhospital settings may thus harbor resentments and fears about domination by a hospital—and its ethics committee.

The third reason to have separate ethics consultation capacity for each type of entity within the organization is that ethics committees should not just advise staff in individual cases; they should also provide ethics education for all staff and employees. They need setting-specific expertise in order to do that properly. A teaching physician who is a wonderful, productive member of an acute-care hospital ethics committee may not be all that useful in providing professional ethics education to a geriatric nurse practitioner who supervises nursing home staff.

Although the education function can, and probably should, be based in an overall organizational ethics body, the actual education must be provided, at least in part, by practitioners who are familiar with the types of ethics problems that arise in the particular setting— be it inpatient, outpatient, longterm, shortterm, or community-based.

Probably the best shortterm solution, then, is to foster the development of specialized ethics consultation capacity that is appropriate to the various elements within the comprehensive organization. This could be in the form of adding expertise to existing committees, establishing subcommittees, or even forming full-blown ethics advisory groups for each entity in the organization.

There should only be one committee for each type of entity— hospital, nursing home, and so forth. To allow every single division to have its own ethics advisory committee is to guarantee turf wars and conflicts for years to come.

3. Establish a coordinating ethics body. Should there be a coordinating ethics body of some kind for the entire organization? I think so, although that may not be a majority view. It just seems to me that although certain ethics functions and needs are specific to the setting, others are organization-wide and require organizational consistency.

One example is the Patient Self-Determination Act, which as of December 1991 required that patients being admitted to a hospital or receiving home healthcare (and some other patients) be informed of the state's laws involving advance directives, such as living wills, and be given the opportunity to execute such documents. But even if this act does not apply to every patient cared for by the organization, it seems silly not to make the same offer to every patient, no matter where he or she makes contact with the organization (even if it is through the group practice or Meals on Wheels).

Another organization-wide need is resource allocation, especially in a capitation environment. Certainly the goal of many integrated healthcare organizations is contracting with employers, insurers, or the government for large numbers of patients in a given region, with capitated payment.

There are a host of ethics issues involved with capitation, including the risks of under-care (we get so involved with watching for the overprovision of services that we forget that capitation arrangements can produce too-skimpy care), competition within the organization for resources, and the relative funding levels of various services.

Furthermore, if the organization really is integrated, then some patients are likely to be moving around from service to service—from acute care to longterm care to homecare, for example. Such patients should be subject to the same ethics policies and rules, no matter which part of the organization is treating them at the moment. That requires overall ethics policies.

Also, some forms of ethics education should be organization-wide, just as some should be service-specific. Examples, in addition to the Patient Self-Determination Act and proper levels of care under capitation, are dealing with HIV-positive patients, confidentiality of patient information, and reporting of improper and unethical conduct. The rules governing such situations should be consistent throughout the organization, and educational activities that promulgate and explain those rules thus should be organization-wide. The best means of ensuring that this comes about is to have an organizational ethics presence, which can be (but does not necessarily have to be) composed of members of the division-specific ethics committees, along with board members of the overall organization. No matter what the chosen structure, trustee involvement is essential.

The rise of integrated organizations that can provide truly comprehensive services to patients on a capitated basis is one of the most welcome and exciting aspects of late-twentieth century healthcare. New, more effective, appropriate ethics structures should be part of their development.

Paradise Lost

A 21st Century Fable

May 1992

It's a privilege to keynote the National Healthcare Ethics and Policy Conference in this year 2000. As you know, this will be the first presidential election since the passage in 1997 of the Universal Healthcare Coverage Act. This law was designed to preserve pluralism, ensure access to care for all Americans, and control costs. The Act required all employers to offer coverage to their workers, expanded Medicaid and Medicare, and provided subsidies to just about everyone: low-income patients, providers, insurers, and some employers.

However, both Amy Carter and Ron Reagan (the major parties' candidates for president) are now criticizing the program, saying it is too complex and expensive and that it gave away the store to providers and insurers. There are also moves in Congress and in state legislatures to repeal the Act.

We are thus seeing a resurgence of enthusiasm for a program similar to that in Canada, where the government is the only payer, institutional providers have global budgets, and physicians negotiate fees with the government. (The same would be true of nurses, who, of course, are widely engaged in autonomous practice.) Several states have applied for waivers from the Universal Healthcare Coverage Act in order to implement such a program.

All this does not portend well for private insurance, an already troubled sector. All Blue Cross and Blue Shield plans, in order to save their tax exemptions, have continued or returned to their original practices of community rating, no medical testing, limits on underwriting and pre-existing condition waiting periods, and open enrollment. But they have paid a price: Bankruptcies among Blue Cross and Blue Shield plans, presaged by the bankruptcy in 1990 of the West Virginia plan, have led to massive federal and state subsidies of most Cross and Shield plans in order to keep them solvent.

Footprints on Your Premium

Meanwhile, a new firm, Health Risk Analysis, Inc., founded by researchers originally funded by the Health Care Financing Administration, has been marketing a computer program that, on the basis of a newborn's footprint, can determine that infant's risk of contracting 47 major diseases in adulthood.

This information, along with the infant's social security number and personal 23-digit ZIP code, is then relayed to a pooled data bank funded by all commercial insurers. When individuals with information in this data bank reach the age of 18 and are eligible for adult coverage under the Act, they will, if they choose commercial insurance, instantly be risk-grouped and their premiums priced accordingly.

The unintended result of this and similar programs, of course, is that although 76 percent of Americans were covered by private insurance in 1989, only 15 percent are privately insured today, and most of them are covered by Blue Cross, Blue Shield, Kaiser-Permanente, or other nonprofit plans. The majority of Americans have public insurance either because they were rejected by commercial insurers or because they could not afford the nonprofits' premiums. Commercial carriers remain in the market largely because all employers are required to offer a commercial alternative, in order to preserve pluralism, and because many receive government subsidies.

The effort to maintain pluralism has doomed cost containment. The per capita cost of coverage is now almost $10,000, and federal subsidies of various healthcare entities now cost more than did the old Medicare and Medicaid programs, which, as you know, were combined in 1996.

No one knows what Congress will do. A Canadian-style plan would be the most moderate of three expected proposals. Another will be Congressman Ron Dellums' bill for a national health service similar to that in Great Britain, where the government owns the hospitals and either employs or contracts with physicians and nurses. This legislation, which was first submitted in the Eighties and was considered radical at the time, now has 85 cosponsors.

The third proposal comes from Minnesota Senator Paul Wellstone, now in his second term. He proposes People's Health Councils, which will be given block grants representing their areas' percentage of national health expenditures. They will distribute these funds as they see fit, after holding town meetings on the subject. Should any of these bills pass—and one of them will—pluralism and private coverage are likely to go the way of microwave ovens, fax machines, car phones, and other fads of the Eighties that are now obsolete.

That is the context within which I have been asked to discuss social ethics issues of this new millennium.

Three Major Dilemmas

I was considering this assignment as I attended the annual meeting of the American Association of Biomedical Ethics Programs (AABEP), held at the new Disney World resort in Moscow. It was attended by 35,000 representatives of the more than 2,000 bioethics centers and programs now extant in the United States. (Given the decline in the number of hospitals to just over 4,000, there is now one bioethics organization for every two hospitals.)

At the AABEP meeting, we identified three major dilemmas in the social ethics of healthcare:

1. How can we guarantee access for all and still keep costs within the limits the government has set on overall healthcare expenditures? Rationing remains an issue, of course, because of the tension between the commitment to universal access and the fact of limited resources. There are those who still argue that healthcare should be funded at the rate of increase it enjoyed between 1970 and 1996—10 to 12 percent a year. When the money runs out, these analysts say, media and public outrage will force more funds out of the government. This way of doing things has prevailed in the United Kingdom for years. But there are doubts that such an approach would work here, because with so many programs and insurers, it would be hard to determine which payers are underfunding the system.

The rationing debate has been discreet, for the most part. There have been some public incidents, of course, such as the publication in the *New England Journal of Medicine* of a major study showing that interleukin-7, at a cost per course of treatment of $150,000, would cure the common cold. As lawsuits filed by patients demanding that insurers cover this cost mounted, a study was published in the *Journal of the American Medical Association*, proving that the findings had been faked by the researchers, who turned out to be heavily invested in a firm that manufactures interleukin-7.

And the organ transplant battles have gone on. As transplantation's effectiveness improved and waiting lists lengthened, "queue-jumping" by patients willing to pay more than prevailing rates was recently exposed on "60 Minutes."

Meanwhile, despite widespread education efforts by community and statewide ethics groups, and despite pleas from state and federal legislators for guidance, public opinion polls continue to show the same inconsistent results: 96 percent of Americans support universal access; 96 percent of Americans believe that access to care should be restricted in some way in order to control costs; 96 percent of Americans believe that people who can afford to buy more care than is required by the Act should be able to do so; and 96 percent of

Americans believe no one should be denied any useful care, even if he or she cannot afford to buy more.

Deep divisions also plague the society in terms of who deserves how much care. Children continue to be viewed as the most meritorious, except for those who have HIV disease or are profoundly disabled; highly politicized debate continues over the level of care that should be provided to them. However, there is no longer much controversy over pediatric liver transplants, despite the fact that the five-year survival rate is only 15 percent, and many of the 200 centers performing the procedure have relatively few patients, leading to even poorer results.

On the other hand, although the Universal Healthcare Coverage Act requires universal immunization of children, millions of young Americans are not protected, as the current measles, tuberculosis, polio, and diphtheria epidemics attest. It is ironic that while poor health status indicators for children helped spur passage of the Act, implementation of its immunization goals does not appear to be a priority.

Public opinion polls reveal that, after children (at least in theory), pregnant women and employed men and women are thought to be the most deserving of care and should be favored in any rationing scheme. But these polls also show that respondents tend to think that the most deserving patients are those most like themselves. Thus white Americans favor whites, black Americans favor blacks, Asians favor Asians, Hispanics favor Hispanics, and so forth.

Indeed, there are widespread reports that physicians and hospitals are ignoring the mandate that they treat all who come to them. Even with universal coverage, low-income patients, people of color, those with HIV disease, and the chronically ill elderly still face compromised access to care. Of course, in New York, where all physicians are now salaried employees of the state, this is not a problem.

Another suggested basis for rationing has been poor health habits. As you know, people whose habits are deemed self-abusive are subject to penalties and co-payments under the Universal Healthcare Coverage Act. This was the result of amendments to the Act sponsored by Senator Jesse Helms, who attached them to the 1997 Consolidated Omnibus Consensual Mostly Agreed to Desperation Budget Reconciliation and Good Riddance Act, which was passed in 1999, long after the fiscal year to which it applied had ended.

Under these amendments, people who do not perform enough sit-ups under federal guidelines, consume more than the suggested liquor allowance, use crack cocaine, fail to wear seat belts, or weigh more than 120 percent of their ideal weight are assessed a surcharge of 20 to 50 percent on their co-payments, depending on whether the arbitration panel—composed of National Football League field officials—believes the offense was intentional or accidental. The Smokers Penalty Amendment, which was bitterly opposed by Senator Helms, was added by the California congressional delegation (which now represents one in four members of Congress), and has the same provisions as the Helms amendments.

A package of amendments designed to expand these penalties to people who use marijuana, starve themselves into anorexia, sustain sports injuries, ski, hang-glide, work more than 12 hours a day, or are dependent on mineral water, oat bran, or other substances recently found addictive is still tied up in a House committee. Members of that committee are currently on a skiing holiday in the Rockies.

2. Is healthcare a public good or a private commodity? This question is entangled with the general debate over whether pluralism in healthcare financing is still the best way to go, or whether a centralized one-payer system is preferable.

The ideological lines have been drawn and the discussion is fiercely partisan, yet it seems clear that the public and private roles of healthcare are inextricably intertwined. Providers claim that government interferes with their practice, but they are quite willing to accept government money, and University of Pennsylvania historian Rosemary Stevens recently testified to Congress that government has provided generous subsidies to many hospitals and physicians almost since the country began. Furthermore, with government now providing 85 percent of all healthcare funds, public payers have adopted the stance that whether healthcare is a public good or not philosophically, it is a public good by default because it is publicly funded.

Some ethics analysts question whether we need to resolve this issue. After all, in this society healthcare is treated as both a commodity and a public service, as both private and public property, and as both a market product and a human service. Perhaps the discussion should focus, not on trying to redefine the roles healthcare plays in society—profit center, luxury, employer, basic right, source of hope, and last resort among them—but rather on the rules we ask providers to follow, in terms of policy, practice, and ethics.

3. What is the responsibility of healthcare providers to society?

Of course, it was widely thought this was all settled with the passage of universal access and requirements that providers accept all patients. But nagging questions remain. For example, after 39 states and the District of Columbia repealed or limited hospital tax exemptions during the late Nineties, debate arose over how hospitals should discharge their social responsibilities. Many states adopted standards based on the 1990 criteria adopted by Utah.

The notorious Utopia Memorial Hospital case of 1998, as you may remember, involved a facility that, weary of trying to meet more and more requirements in order to keep its tax exemption, decided to convert to for-profit status. It was promptly sued by its home state for $50 million in back taxes. The state argued that if the hospital had conceded its *de facto* profit-oriented status all along, the state would have been able to collect taxes from it. The resulting bankruptcy of the hospital put an end to similar efforts by other institutions.

There are other issues involving the social role of hospitals and physicians. One is their responsibility in death and dying, which has been brought to the fore by the ballot initiative in Massachu-setts that seeks to require any provider to assist any patient in com-mitting suicide, no matter what the situation. In the wake of the 1990 Cruzan decision by the US Supreme Court, the public has become so frightened that patients will not be able to end unwanted treatment that the initiative is expected to pass overwhelmingly.

Given the 1992 conviction for murder in Michigan of patholo-gist Jack Kevorkian, who despite many warnings continued to enable patient suicides in his van in various parks in the state, providers are left between a rock and hard place in terms of issues of suicide and termination of treatment. However, a survey con-ducted in 1999 by the Joint Commission on Accreditation of Every-thing in Healthcare (JCAEH) found that those healthcare organizations and physicians with clear, explicit policies on termi-nation of treatment and patient preference, which were routinely shared with patients, had virtually no litigation.

But the overriding issue in terms of provider social responsi-bility involves who it is that they purport to serve. This began with revelations in 1990 that there were four times as many mam-mography machines in the United States as would be needed if every woman in the country were receiving the procedure at rec-ommended intervals. Because of the resulting low volume, the cost of mammography had increased rather than decreased in the face of oversupply.

Yet the rate of mortality from breast cancer among low-income women was rising, largely because of lack of early detection. Ques-tions were thus raised about whether the healthcare system was con-figured to benefit patients—whom providers claimed they served—or providers, who had received most of the benefit.

With rates of immunization and prenatal care plummeting, not because of lack of payment but because of provider disinterest; with fewer people choosing medicine as a career because medical school faculty members insist on mourning the good old days rather than sparking enthusiasm for the future; and with healthcare system overcapacity a scandal, opinion polls show that the public thinks the healthcare system has enriched itself at the expense of patients, and has tried to force patients to accommodate to its wants.

There were portents of all this. George Lundberg, MD, the editor of the *Journal of the American Medical Association*, wrote in an editorial in January 1990 that the business side of medicine was eclipsing the professional and ethical side, to the detriment of the profession. He wrote that medicine, "up to and into the next millennium, must be obviously in the public interest and of worldwide scope. It must ensure access to care of acceptable quality for all, practice economic soundness, balance health fairly against all other societal needs, emphasize good communications, and most of all require and demonstrate good will toward all people. By so doing, we can preserve our profession into the next millennium for future generations of physicians." In response, at the 1990 AMA annual meeting, some delegates called for his resignation. He was fired in 1996, of course, after his public condemnation of the physicians and hospitals who organized the Association to Refuse Care to HIV Patients, but his editorial lived on. And, as you know, last year he won the Nobel Prize for Medicine.

Similarly, the late David Kinzer of Harvard University had pointed out in *Hospitals* in April 1988 that hospital administrators had given a standing ovation to a Reagan Administration representative in 1981 who had said that healthcare funding must be cut in order to build up the defense budget. Kinzer observed, "This outburst seemed to break one of the rules in our field—that if you don't care about what happens to the sick poor, you should at least keep quiet about it."

But hospitals did not, and by the end of the Eighties, they had neither their autonomy nor the money to care for the sick poor who were still in their laps. Kinzer's admonition: "I suggest that if the next administration announces plans for more retrenchment, it would be best not to stand up and cheer." But delegates to the 1992

AHA annual meeting gave Congressman Newt Gingrich a standing ovation when he did just that.

As I survey the proposed legislation in this year 2000, it doesn't
look good. Clearly, we are seeing the end of a private, pluralistic system; the best we can hope for is a Canadian-style approach. The
commercial insurers and the Blues could well cease to exist during
this congressional session.

The patient-provider relationship, already shaky, is likely to be
tightly defined by legislation and regulation in terms of which treatment to choose, where the patient will be treated, termination of
care, and quality of death; physicians and patients will have little
say in the matter. Patients who are subjects of biomedical research,
of course, are already directly monitored by the federal government,
as a result of the informed consent scandals of the mid-Nineties.

Tax policy will be used to manipulate nonprofit hospitals and
insurers (if they survive). The massive capital indebtedness of the
for-profits, whose patients are few and far between in this age of
mandatory prospective review of all admissions, is likely to doom
most of them to bankruptcy, although some will eke out an existence
providing liposuction, weight-loss counseling, and cosmetic surgery.

This all came about, it appears, because people stopped trusting
providers. Healthcare could have remained an honorable, trusted,
ethical component of society, but it chose not to, believing instead
that it could indulge in endless excess without getting caught. And
so it gave away the priceless privilege of defining its own ethics.

This did not have to happen.

. . . .

*This column is based on remarks originally presented at the Estes
Park Institute National Hospital Medical Staff-Trustee Conference, Kona, Hawaii, January 1991.*

As Long As It Comes Out All Right

July 1992

One of my favorite sayings is: "Be careful what you wish for; you might get it." It certainly has its applications in healthcare. Indeed, for those of us who have been advocating the use of outcomes data and comparative measures of treatment options in the evaluation of the quality and efficacy of care, the coming of real commitment to outcomes-based assessment is most welcome—but almost surprising after all this time. After all, one of the first advocates of the use of outcomes data was Florence Nightingale, and the pioneering work of John Wennberg, MD, and his colleagues on variations in medical practice patterns began during the late Sixties. For that matter, I wrote my first ethics column in this journal about the use of health services research data in 1987!

Despite my enthusiasm for placing the provision and evaluation of care on a more objective, scientific, and patient-oriented basis, I must add a cautionary note. Certain parts of the outcomes revolution hold the potential for leaving me sorry that I wished for it.

So, even as the outcomes drumbeats grow louder, I want to bring up a few issues of ethical concern in connection with the use of outcomes as a basis for quality evaluation and provider payment.

Knee-Jerk Interpretation

In December 1991, pursuant to a suit filed by *Newsday* under the Freedom of Information Act, the names of 140 physicians in New

York state who performed coronary artery bypass grafts were released to the public, accompanied by the adjusted mortality rate for each physician's patients.

Two findings were notable: First, mortality rates varied even among physicians working at the same hospital, which probably wasn't much of a surprise to anyone familiar with the data on variations in physician practice patterns. Second, physicians who performed fewer than the 50 bypass operations a year recommended as a minimum threshold by a state advisory committee had higher mortality rates than physicians who performed more than 50. This, too, is not a shock. The relationship of higher volume to lower mortality for cardiac procedures was established for hospitals years ago, and was expected to hold true for physicians.

Consumer advocates argued successfully that the public has a right to know the track records of physicians doing risky surgery. It's certainly a persuasive argument. But did anyone have a thought for the physicians whose reputations, vulnerability to malpractice suits, and hospital privileges could be put at risk by the release of this information? Would anyone like to argue that we know and understand all the hundreds of factors that produce a given outcome, and that they were all taken into consideration and the data adjusted accordingly before this information was released? I doubt it.

So certain surgeons in New York state who might be reliable, good practitioners have now been portrayed in the press as having poor outcomes, with the implication that their competence is questionable. Likewise, certain surgeons whose patient mortality rates are low and whose outcomes appear great may not, in fact, be the best in the business.

In a classic essay on outcomes, Steven Schroeder, MD, now president of the Robert Wood Johnson Foundation, pointed out that apparent bad outcomes—even mortality, which in most cases is about as bad an outcome as one can have—do not necessarily mean poor performance. He cautioned against cavalier interpretation of outcomes data, warning that "after all, the best outcomes from elective surgery would be observed with healthy patients who may not even have needed the operation."

We need to go beyond adjustments for age, gender, diagnosis, and severity of illness (and we have hardly perfected methodologies for assessing the latter, despite what research entrepreneurs claim) to more subtle issues such as the patient's nutritional status, psychological state (was she depressed?), family situation, "social severity" (low-income and other disadvantaged patients often have worse outcomes, regardless of other variables), and other factors.

An example: In one smallish state that has a statewide hospital database, the largest and most prestigious teaching hospital in the state showed up with the worst mortality rates for a broad range of conditions. Did this mean it was a terrible hospital? No, it probably meant that the referral network designed to send the sickest and most complicated cases to that hospital was working. I'd feel a lot less confident in that network if a small primary care hospital in a thinly populated rural area had the worst mortality rates!

It's similar to the situation that arose when a study was published showing that "regulation" (defined, oddly, as control of the hospital bed supply) was associated with higher rates of death in hospitals—that is, when the bed supply was tight and occupancy high, mortality rates in hospitals were higher. A health economist of my acquaintance remarked about the study, "That means if hospital beds are in short supply, sicker people occupy them. That is what *should* happen!"

All this is to say that outcomes information is still pretty fuzzy stuff, and I don't think we can make exaggerated claims for its validity any more than we can dismiss it as useless. We are in a middle ground here, and our ethical responsibility is to release, interpret, and use outcomes data within the limits of what is appropriate and reasonable.

That is a very difficult chore for the public press, especially the broadcast press, who have a minute or two to tell the story, and can hardly resort to the use of footnotes to caution against jumping to conclusions. Healthcare researchers and providers need to help them do that job better.

But providers can be just as sloppy as the media in using outcomes information, especially if it makes the provider look good. We have already seen hospitals use mortality rates in advertisements because the rates appeared to make them look good. Yet we can rest assured that if the mortality rates had made them look bad, those same hospitals would be screaming bloody murder.

As we move to physician-specific outcomes information, I'm afraid we can expect more expose-type coverage in the public press, more irresponsible advertising by hospitals and physicians, and inappropriate use of outcomes data in the granting of privileges and the credentialing of physicians. This could make "economic credentialing"— a moral swamp in itself—look like a sane, rational, scientific process.

Confidentiality

This is a very challenging issue. If, for example, outcomes studies consistently show a given physician, hospital, or HMO to have poor results, it's not going to protect anyone to keep the information confidential or to release it without the names of the perpetrators attached.

On the other hand, my reaction to the New York release of physicians' names was one of great discomfiture. Some of these surgeons' practices could be lost and their lives ruined while, three years down the line, new research could show that their high mortality rates could be easily justified. To quote Leon Wyszewianski, one of the clearest thinkers in this field, "Most of us are fated to die despite the best of care."

Furthermore, two pioneering programs in use of outcomes data to change physician and hospital practice—the Maryland Hospital Association's Quality Indicators Project and the Maine Medical Assessment Foundation—have operated just fine while keeping data confidential. In both cases, the assumption is that providers are more likely to learn, and to change, if they are not in the paranoid

....

position of being threatened with "exposure" of questionable practice patterns and results.

However, there is a very tough tradeoff here that both ethics and the Hippocratic Oath ("do no harm") require: If the names of providers (individual or institutional) whose track records are questionable are to be kept confidential, then the healthcare field itself must have policies and procedures for protecting patients that are as tough as can be—no exceptions for high admitters, no reprieves for repeat offenders, no giving of passes to those who are impaired or financially strapped.

For example, the Joint Commission on Accreditation of Healthcare Organizations last year was forced to disaccredit Cook County Hospital, one of the most-needed facilities in the city of Chicago, if not the nation. This was not done lightly. (The hospital has since regained its accreditation.) Similarly, some public hospitals in New York state have not fared well in mortality rate studies. This may well be due to the "social severity" of their patients—I would be surprised if it were not—but if it turns out to be a problem of persistent poor quality, then their patients must be protected.

Keep in mind that it was the failure of providers to act on blatant information about poor quality—physicians who raped or mutilated patients, unnecessary care, HMOs skimping on needed services—that led journalists and consumer advocates to demand the public release of healthcare data. If we wish to protect providers from the inappropriate release or interpretation of outcomes data, we had better have internal mechanisms for protecting patients that will stand up to anyone's scrutiny. So far, we don't have them, and even when we do, we don't use them.

Who Is Responsible for Improvement?

Healthcare providers right now are enamored with the continuous quality improvement/total quality management idea. With the coming of useful outcomes data, however, the idea of continuing to improve quality within an organization runs into the idea that regulators, payers, consumer groups, and other entities will be using outcomes data to compare performance between organizations. And may the "best" hospital win!

Given that the "competitive ethic" (which more and more is looking like a contradiction in terms) feeds the idea that the highest-quality provider will prevail, the use of comparative outcomes data threatens to create a nightmarish situation in which those providers who can manipulate patient mix, medical staff, and data best can get all the managed care and Medicare contracts—and all the other hospitals, physicians, and HMOs whose data don't measure up can go bankrupt.

What gets lost here is a basic question: Is quality assessment supposed to let some providers win and others lose, or should it improve the performance of the entire provider community? In other words, if St. Anywhere Hospital has poor outcomes, do we simply give all the business to Memorial instead and throw St. Anywhere (and its patients) to the dogs? Remember that in economic theory, the endpoint, the ultimate goal, of competition is monopoly. Is that what we want?

What if St. Anywhere's patients include large numbers of destitute homeless people, poor minority people with HIV disease, frail elderly women with multiple morbidities, and cocaine-addicted teenage mothers? Did the outcomes studies reflect that? And will Memorial Hospital graciously take on these patients, whom until now it has assiduously avoided?

More and more studies are showing that certain patient groups, such as those just noted, have trouble getting care no matter what their insurance status. And maybe Memorial's data look good because Memorial doesn't deal with tough cases like these, which involve a range of social problems not directly reflected in clinical data. Where does the outcomes movement leave them?

Outcomes data, if they are to be a meaningful part of the movement toward continuous quality improvement, must be seen as markers along the road that point the direction in which we need to go. They cannot be seen as endpoints that determine the winners and losers, whether within an organization or within a community. Otherwise the "improvement" part of the equation becomes an exercise in hypocrisy.

Conflict of Interest

All those of you who think that outcomes data will not be used to determine payment, raise your hands. Those of you who did, see me later; I have some Texas savings and loan stock I would like to sell you, cheap.

It is not a coincidence that major payers like Medicare, large employers, Blue Cross and Blue Shield, and Aetna are heavily involved in the use of severity adjustment methodologies and software for measuring the "appropriateness" of care. The federal government has promulgated guidelines for treatment of post-surgical pain and urinary incontinence, and several payers have established standards for the use of cesarean section, some of which are tied to reimbursement. Very clearly, payment will be on the basis of outcomes, and quite soon.

The problem here is one of conflict of interest. A payer who determines the acceptability of the outcome of a procedure or test for which it is also paying will have something of a bias (to put it mildly) to use outcomes standards that favor conservative, less expensive care. Now, I, for one, believe that in most cases, conservative care that happens to be less expensive is probably better care. However, I fear the institutionalization of that philosophy, especially when it comes to managed care, because of the threat that we will shift from overcare to undercare without passing "GO" or collecting $200. I particularly fear it when the decision is in the hands of payers, who are not exactly going to have the objectivity of Solomon, regardless of what methods or tools they are using.

Years ago, Dr. Wennberg pointed out that when rates vary, there is no scientific basis for automatically assuming that any rate—high, low, or middle—is the appropriate rate of use for that procedure. The key, he concluded, would be the results associated with each rate. He was, and is, entirely correct. But if a payer will greatly benefit by assuming that the lowest rate is right, then patients will be as much at risk as they were when providers assumed that "the more, the merrier" was the high-quality way to go.

My father, who is a pathologist, rarely seeks healthcare. When I asked him why, he replied, "Pathologists are therapeutic nihilists." And indeed, given that pathologists are confronted disproportionately with the bodies of patients who did not survive, whose treatments did not work, whose care did not save them, therapeutic nihilism seems a logical stance for them. However, it is a dangerous stance for payers, and one that cannot be allowed to prevail unchecked.

Profiteering

After International Medical Centers, a notorious Florida Medicare HMO with powerful political connections to the Reagan-Bush administration and a habit of undertreating its patients, was finally exposed and put out of business, a few of us asked another basic question: If you can make more money keeping people away from care than you can providing care, won't the venture capitalists, entrepreneurs, and profiteers head in that direction?

The answer is: Did they ever! Today, researchers patent products that were developed with taxpayers' or tax-exempt foundation money, and make millions selling them to employers and payers. Severity systems, outcomes systems, utilization review systems, "appropriateness" systems—millions are being made.

A private utilization review firm recently bought itself another firm that owned a couple of HMOs and other holdings for $100 million. Placement of some severity systems can cost $100,000 per setting. The field is rife with "black-box" products whose methodologies, measures, and processes are trade secrets. And we wonder why physicians resist being evaluated by such tools!

Uwe Reinhardt of Princeton University once said that the venture capitalists came to healthcare because there was basically nowhere else in the economy for them to go. It is not surprising that they are now forging into the outcomes field, cannibalizing methods and databases, developing their private little systems, peddling their wares to payers, and laughing all the way to the bank. Meanwhile, 40 million people have no health insurance, and our children continue to die of measles.

I have no love of healthcare profiteering. When a hospital with $100 million in the bank announces that it can no longer "afford" to provide emergency services to the uninsured poor, I stand with the government: Tax its profits, because they are profits, and they are not being used for community benefit. When a physician makes a seven-figure income providing liposuction or breast augmentation to women whose self-image has been eroded by an unforgiving society, I am sickened.

But I am no less sickened by "quality" experts and "outcomes managers" and consultants who gleefully explain to the powers that be how even needed care can be denied, choice compromised, and patients' interests overlooked—for a fee that would immunize every child in the community and then some. And heaven forfend that these gurus provide *pro bono* service to a struggling county hospital or community clinic!

I must repeat: The coming of outcomes-based quality assessment is one of the most important and welcome developments in healthcare in the late 20th century. I believe it can lead to more scientific medicine, more appropriate care, healthier patients, and better providers—if we do it right.

But if we are sloppy or greedy or unthinking or self-serving in implementing these concepts, the damage we do will come back to haunt us. For the unethical use of outcomes information can lead, not to enhanced results, but to the poorest of poor care.

A Matter of Principle

September 1992

*This was the first of three columns on healthcare
reform (the other two, also in this volume, were
"Freedom of Choice" and "Losers"). None of what
I and many other people had hoped for came to pass;
the prediction is now that 60 million or more Americans will be uninsured by the turn of the century.
What a swell way to start the third millennium.*

In the past year, and especially the past few months, we have seen
health policy take more and more of a central role in our political debates—after years of intentional (and destructive) neglect.

Three more states—Florida, Minnesota, and Vermont—have
joined the list of those that have passed laws intended to provide
universal coverage of healthcare costs. (Hawaii has already done so,
as did Massachusetts, although the latter law has not been fully
implemented and probably never will be, in its present form.) The
pile of healthcare reform proposals in Congress has never been fat-
ter, even though there is not much optimism that anything of substance will pass before the election.

In Pennsylvania, appointed incumbent Senator Harris Wofford,
a Democrat, defeated supposedly popular ex-governor Richard
Thornburgh for the seat of the late Senator John Heinz, a Republican. Wofford ran on a platform of vague promises about universal

health insurance. Many other candidates for state and national office have taken up the issue, and even President George Bush, who had shown little interest in health policy, unveiled a health-care reform proposal, although the only legislation it has produced is a bill proposing some mild private insurance market reforms.

"Sound and Fury, Signifying Nothing"

I, for one, am pleased by some aspects of this. Issues such as equity, quality of care, healthcare human resource availability and distribution, affordability, and access to needed and timely care are very important to me.

But health policy and health politics are two different things. And while there is action aplenty in Congress and state legislatures, I am reminded of the words of Macbeth upon his being told that his wife is dead. He describes life as "a tale told by an idiot, full of sound and fury, signifying nothing."

For every Minnesota, where something meaningful has been done, there is a California, where healthcare reform has inspired an enormous amount of squabbling, name-calling, and noise, but nothing has been done. Indeed, the healthcare reform initiative that will be on the California ballot in November could actually retard progress on the issue, perhaps for years.

In Congress, the Democrats are so busy fighting each other over which healthcare reform proposal they should support (much of which has to do with turf fights among various committee chairmen) that they don't have time to fight with the Republicans, who are less than unified in their efforts, anyway.

Even what should be the rather mundane process of granting waivers to states for experimental programs (whether the radical proposal from Oregon, which I find immoral, or basic requests for traditional Medicaid waivers) has become highly politicized, with ideological posturing at every turn. Partisanship has poisoned the waters to such a degree that no one wants to drink at the health policy waterhole.

It reminds me of the recent era in Australia, when every time the Labor Party got into power, it pushed for universal health insurance; every time the Liberals (which is the conservative party in Australia—don't ask me . . .) got into power, they cut back on universal coverage. As a result, the entire basis of healthcare coverage in Australia was at risk of changing every few years. I asked a planner for a hospital in Melbourne what effect this had on his work, and he just glared at me.

A Proposal

Now we have an election looming, and as the campaigns heat up and I see even basic healthcare issues being kicked around as political footballs, I would like to make a proposal.

It has been noted to the point of overkill that only the United States and South Africa, among developed nations, have not committed themselves to universal access to healthcare for all their citizens. (And who knows? If the South Africans can get back to the bargaining table, and if the Kaiser Family Foundation continues to help them redesign their healthcare system, they may get there before we do.)

What is not usually noted, when it comes to international comparisons, is that most developed nations have also taken basic principles of health policy out of the realm of partisan politics.

Margaret Thatcher, when she was prime minister of Great Britain, would have dearly loved to privatize the socialized National Health Service. She sold off many other nationalized industries and services, but all she could do was nibble around the edges of the NHS (and egregiously underfund it). Brian Mulroney, the conservative prime minister of Canada, faced a firestorm when it was suggested that the free trade agreement between his nation and ours might compromise the Canadian universal health insurance scheme; the uproar was the only serious threat to the treaty. And I was told recently that even the Australian conservatives have now agreed to preserve that nation's universal coverage program, should they come to power.

Other nations have done something very sensible: They have agreed on certain basic principles for the organization, delivery, accessibility, and financing of healthcare services, and declared that those principles should hold regardless of who is in office. In effect, they have put health policy in the same position as our Federal Reserve Board or Supreme Court.

This does not mean that health policies must be frozen in a certain form, or that flexibility in making decisions is lost. It means, as was pointed out recently at a healthcare conference in Montana by Joe Chouinard, director of corporate affairs for the Canadian Medical Association, that the society as a whole agrees on certain values that should guide health policy, and those values are held inviolate.

For example, in Canada five basic principles guide the healthcare system: public administration, universality, accessibility, affordability, and portability. That leaves a lot of wiggle room, and each province does its own thing within those standards. But it means that every Canadian has coverage through a publicly administered plan that will allow him or her accessible care at a reasonable price (in most provinces, with no direct payment by the citizen) and that no matter where in Canada he or she travels or moves to, the coverage will be effective.

Because of all the politics around the Canadian system, let me state categorically that I am not advocating that the United States adopt that particular model. We don't like public administration; furthermore, our healthcare system is mostly private, and there seems to be general agreement that we want to keep it that way. So at least one of the Canadian principles—public administration—would be a no-go here. I am simply using Canada's guiding values as an example of what I would like to see here: political agreement on a set of principles to guide our healthcare system that would be accepted and respected by all, no matter who the changing winds of politics might blow into or out of office.

So, as the election gets closer, I would like to propose my own set of guiding principles for a healthcare system. And by principles, I mean values: the underlying philosophy that guides policy decisions.

1. Universality. Our nation is a very pick-and-choose society; we segregate, we pass judgment, we differentiate. We still try to distinguish between the "deserving" and the "undeserving" poor, and the toxin of racism is everywhere. We simply do not think in terms of all of us being in anything together.

But when it comes to access to healthcare, we have to include everyone: criminals, dope dealers, smokers, hang-gliders, the homeless, the mad, everybody. Otherwise we will simply end up with Medicaid again, which is to say that every time the budgets get tight, we will start tossing powerless people out of the system. That has not worked well for us. So, in terms of the guarantee of access, it must be universal. This also means that a certain level of benefits should be available to everyone, and it should not be a skimpy package.

2. Reasonable access. Universal coverage means nothing if there are no healthcare providers around, or there are healthcare providers around, but they don't like your insurance, your diagnosis, or your looks. We need both coverage and access, which means that providers other than physicians may be needed in underserved areas to deliver primary care, or that better transportation to services will be needed in some areas, or that services may need to go to patients in some areas.

If a person chooses to live in the wilds of Alaska, 200 miles from a town, he or she cannot expect that a university teaching hospital will be established out there to guarantee instant access to all tertiary services. But reasonable access to most healthcare services should be available.

3. Cost containment. Healthcare in the United States costs too much for what we are getting from it. And if it continues to escalate in cost at the rate it has been, no program for coverage or access will be able to survive. Therefore, we must limit costs and their rate of inflation, and we must do so as a society, rather than flailing around as a fragmented series of individual employers, coalitions, third-party payers, and governments, each trying to limit its costs by slipping the bill to someone else. As Howard Dean, MD, the physician-governor of Vermont, recently observed, if you provide insurance with a $5,000 deductible to a person whose annual income is $16,000, you aren't providing insurance.

4. Appropriate, necessary, and timely care. Available healthcare services (I think all healthcare services, but certainly all services that are in any way funded with tax dollars, directly or indirectly) should be limited to those that are needed, and should be provided in the appropriate setting on a timely basis.

That is to say, shutting people out of the system until they are dying and then providing last-minute care in an emergency department is not only immoral, but illogical and wasteful. So is enrolling people in managed care programs that control access to the point that patients can't get care when they need it. We need standards and guidelines for when care is indicated, appropriate settings for the care of given conditions, and timely access. If we did this, we would save enough money to buy first-class health insurance for all the uninsured people in the entire country.

5. Pluralism and competition within reason. Given what I know of American healthcare history and culture, we would prefer a system that gives us as many choices as possible. That does not mean that we really need 1,500 third-party payers and several thousand employers, each paying for other people's healthcare.

But it does mean that in most markets, having several plans available, preferably from several payers, is the most culturally comfortable way for us to go. Also, we are a capitalistic society; therefore, competition should be allowed, as long as it is on the basis of service and effectiveness, not on how viciously a payer can underwrite sick people out of the system or skimp on benefits.

6. As much autonomy as possible for patients and providers alike. To the degree that a system can keep payers out of the physician-patient and hospital-patient relationships, it should do so. I have never been comfortable with the idea of ABC Insurance Company hiring a clerk to sit at a computer to run a program that will dictate a physician's clinical decisions. Let us macro-manage the budgets and stop micro-managing the process of care.

Likewise, the revolution that is taking place in terms of providing patients with clinical information, empowering patients to make treatment decisions, and allowing patients and their loved ones to determine when treatment should be ended and how and when death should occur, must be allowed to continue.

7. Privacy, confidentiality, and respect. The large databases we are developing, the computerized medical record that is going to be a standard tool, the easy availability of information within large managed care organizations, the Freedom of Information Act, the ability of the plaintiff's bar to gather sensitive information for malpractice cases, the coming of genetic testing for hundreds of conditions—these are all threats to the privacy of the healthcare transaction and the dignity of the individual. Americans fail to realize that one does not need the intrusions of government to erode privacy and individuality; all one needs is a computer.

Remember that a healthcare worker snapped a picture of John Lennon's corpse as it was about to be cremated and sold the photo to a tabloid newspaper. The equivalent of that goes on every day with the most personal of information about patients. We need to have more respect for information and the people it concerns.

8. A sense of community. Yes, folks, we are all in this together. To quote Bertrand Russell: "Mankind has become so much one family that we cannot ensure our own prosperity except by ensuring that of everyone else." Therefore, our healthcare system should be based on a belief that everybody ought to be willing to give up something in order to make things better for all of us as a group.

Some states, such as Mississippi, are so poor that they can only enact reforms with outside financial help; that means there must be transfers of resources—of money—between states. Also, Vermont, with a high income tax, must be getting pretty tired of subsidizing New Hampshire and Texas, which have none.

We may need to tax the money made on liposuction, cosmetic surgery, dental phobia clinics, pet psychiatry, and the like in order to fund core services for the disadvantaged. We may need to rein in the excesses of the private boutique psychiatric industry (and that is an industry) in order to do something about the masses of untreated, desperately mentally ill people living on our streets.

We will need to reorder our priorities. And that is going to gore everyone's ox, at least a little. It will be a lot less painful if we dust off what was once a key American value, and accept that it is a good thing to give to the less fortunate, especially if you have a whole lot more than they do.

Do Vote

These principles/values may sound utopian when viewed against the often polluted backdrop of American politics, but that does not mean they are irrelevant. I would hope that you would at least keep them in mind when you go to vote.

And do vote. Know where you want health policy to go, and vote for those who want to go there, too. If you do not, you have no right to complain if the health policy gridlock continues.

The Littlest Victims

November 1992

It was 1969. I was working nights, weekends, and holidays at a hospital in California. I delivered lab slips. One of my stops was the pediatric department, where one day a beautiful little girl was admitted with head injuries. I believe her parents said she had fallen. She was treated, kept for observation, and released. She was back a few days later, with more injuries. Another excuse was given. She was released to her parents. The revolving door continued, with admissions and releases, until her last admission. This time she was dead.

Another time, I watched the rage of a nurse as she debrided burns on the feet of an infant who had been forced to stand in scalding hot water. I felt helpless, and so did she.

Good health, according to the World Health Organization, is not simply the absence of illness, but is rather the presence of well-being, including good physical and mental health, nutrition, housing, and a stable family and social environment. Good healthcare, then, is more than treatment of symptoms; it should include treatment of causes. Judged by this standard, one of our healthcare system's greatest failures has been in the area of child abuse. We have not only failed to prevent it; in some ways we have actually aided this society as it abandoned the littlest victims of cruelty.

It is certainly not a new phenomenon. Among people I have encountered in my life are a woman whose parents told her they were tired of her and left her at an orphanage; a woman who was repeatedly raped by her father; a woman whose going-away gift, when she went off to college as an honor student, was a black eye; a man whose parents kept him locked in a closet for most of his childhood, letting him out only to attend school; and a spectacularly beautiful woman whose father insisted for all of his days that she was ugly beyond belief.

Those are people I have met or known personally. They do not include Johnny Lindquist, who was hung from a rope and used as a punching bag by his father until he died; Lindsey Murdock, raped and murdered by a stranger who left him to die under a pile of garbage; a Chicago boy who was gang-raped over a period of months by neighbor boys; the infant whose parents fed him sulfuric acid; Oprah Winfrey, the television star, sexually abused by an uncle; Marilyn Van Derbur, former Miss America, raped for years by her father; writer Maya Angelou, raped as a child and so traumatized by the event and its aftermath that she did not speak a word for years; or Lisa Steinberg, the illegally adopted daughter of an upscale New York City attorney who beat her to death.

I should add Charles Manson and a number of other serial killers, all of whom, a recent study concluded, were victims of child abuse and neglect. So strong is the association between mistreatment in childhood and the committing of multiple murders in adulthood that one psychologist, an expert in profiling serial killers, had a chilling answer when he was asked the one thing we should do to stop more such murderers from emerging: "We should stop torturing our children."

Hopes Strangled

These are the dramatic cases, the ones we hear about. They mask the millions of children whose self-esteem is destroyed, self-confidence butchered, hopes strangled, and futures dimmed by emotional abuse—unrelenting attacks of parents or others on a child's very identity. When the people who are supposed to protect you and take pride in you instead teach you to hate yourself, where can you hide? As one victim of hideous emotional abuse told me, "Sometimes I think physical abuse is better; at least it stops at some point. The emotional attacks just go on and on."

One of the most common statements made by people who were emotionally or physically abused as children is, "I wasn't sexually abused." Hidden in those tragic words is the unstated belief, so common among the abused, that it could have been worse, so maybe it wasn't so bad. Also hidden there is the private guilt of the abused, the almost universal belief, pounded into them, that somehow it was their fault.

Am I overdoing it? Is this making you uncomfortable? Consider the following: At the Ninth International Congress on Child Abuse and Neglect in Chicago earlier this year, the National Committee for Prevention of Child Abuse (NCPCA) provided a report noting that 1,383 American children died of child abuse and neglect in 1991, a 10.3 percent increase over the previous year.

An estimated 2,694,000 children were reported to child protection agencies to be victims of mistreatment. Data from 21 states indicate that 48 percent of cases involved neglect, 25 percent physical abuse, 15 percent sexual abuse, 6 percent emotional abuse, and 10 percent "other" situations. These are considered to be low estimates, because so much abuse of children goes unreported.

On the Front Lines

Healthcare professionals have been more involved in protecting children in recent years. Healthcare facilities and practitioners constitute a front line of defense, charged as they are with reporting suspected mistreatment. They also provide millions of dollars in care for children whose illnesses and injuries are the product of abuse. And some provider groups, such as the American Academy of Pediatrics, have been fervent advocates for children.

Others have developed model programs to prevent abuse. The Hawaii Healthy Start program, through which families that are at high risk of child abuse are identified and supported with home visits and counseling, was highlighted at the international congress for its success. In a group of families identified as high-risk, 9 percent of children were reported as having encountered mistreatment; only 4 percent of Healthy Start clients were reportedly abused.

But we are not doing enough, in either the microcosm of the individual care encounter or the macrocosm of public policy.

For one thing, the reporting of abuse after the fact only protects children from future harm (sometimes); and in many states, the crushing overload on caseworkers and the tendency to return children to abusive family situations often mean it doesn't even do that. Shortages of foster families, funds, and staffing for alternative living situations, not only for children but also for their battered parents, hardly helps the situation.

Furthermore, much abuse is not reported. Some of this is the result of the victims being terrified of telling anyone about what is going on; abusive behavior is often accompanied by threats of dire consequences if the victim tells. Some of it is the increasing and tragic tendency of people in this country not to "get involved," especially if there is a threat of retaliation from the abuser. If you believe that a lawsuit, harassment, or even physical danger will be the result of your reporting abuse, you will be far more hesitant to do so.

But some of it has to do with the fact that providers are quite capricious in what they do and do not report. One of the ironies of the Lisa Steinberg case was the consternation expressed by the press that a well-to-do attorney was a child abuser; this seems to have been a surprise. It should not have been; child abuse is hardly the exclusive province of the poor.

That poverty and economic stress play a part is incontestable; so is the role of substance abuse. The NCPCA report found that alcohol and drug use was one of the two most common contributing factors. The next most common was poverty or "increased financial stress due to unemployment and the recession."

Providers, however, are far more likely to report low-income parents and people of color as child abusers. In his landmark study (published in the April 26, 1990, *New England Journal of Medicine*), Ira Chasnoff, MD, reported on drug and alcohol use among pregnant women in Pinellas County, Florida, where providers are required to report to health authorities any woman known to be using drugs or alcohol during pregnancy. Although the incidence of drug and alcohol use was similar for white women (15.4 percent) and Black women (14.1 percent), Chasnoff found that Black women were ten times more likely to be reported to authorities, and low-income women were also more likely to be reported.

There are all kinds of possible reasons for these findings, but they also reflect what has been found in other studies: Providers will look the other way when it comes to some patients. It is ironic indeed that although a host of research studies have shown that poor people and people of color, including children, have less access to care regardless of their insurance status, the healthcare community is much more willing to report them for child abuse and neglect.

The other troubling issue with reporting is simply that it involves very, very serious charges; nothing can ruin a person's life as quickly as being accused of child abuse. And if we tend to shy away from reporting some cases because they involve the lifestyles of the rich and famous, we also may be too quick to report others who are not abusers. Certainly the recent flood of highly publicized divorce and palimony cases in which accusations of child abuse have flown from both sides illustrate that such accusations can be very damaging weapons. Enough questions have been raised in some cases to lead most of us to conclude that there are people in jail for abuse who probably did not commit the crime; in some instances, they have lost or are losing their children. And even if they are vindicated, the scars left by the battle can be crippling for them.

We have not done a good enough job of developing reliable means of determining the presence of abuse, and we have done a horrible job of finding ways to prevent it by intervening early. One reason the Hawaii program has been so successful, I think, is that it offers support, counseling, and education, as opposed to the punitive approach illustrated by attempts in Florida and Illinois to jail pregnant, addicted women. Fat lot of good that does anyone!

As long as the healthcare provider is the most likely source of reporting, and the most likely person or entity to whom abused and abuser alike will turn for help, providers must be better educated about abuse, and be given better tools with which to confront it. In the words of Dr. Chasnoff and his colleagues, "If legally mandated reporting is to be free of racial or economic bias, it must be based on objective medical criteria."

Blood on Our Hands

As for public policy, we are all guilty of abuse and neglect. There is blood on all our hands. For we have tolerated and even supported policies that terrorize, maim, and kill children—and we have done so with gusto. This societal child abuse has been manifested in at least five ways:

1. Increased poverty. The Census Bureau reported earlier this year that 35 million Americans now live in poverty, with 2 million more having joined those troubled ranks last year. At least 7.7 million families live in poverty. One-fifth of all American children were in families with incomes below the poverty line in 1989; with the erosion of the economy, that figure is higher now, perhaps one in four.

Poverty hurts children in two ways. First, as noted, poverty is one of the two most common contributing factors in child abuse. Second, poverty has a host of destructive companions: malnutrition, depression, illness, medical indigence, drugs and alcohol, gangs, loss of self-esteem.

Ours is one of the few developed nations on earth that does not seek to guarantee a basic level of protection—food, clothing, housing, medical care, education—to all its children. As a result, it is not just our dreadful rate of infant mortality that should make us hang our heads; it is how we force so many of our children to live.

2. Intergenerational equity. By this I do not mean the vicious argument, promulgated by too many policy dilettantes, that the only way to protect children is to take benefits away from the elderly. (Tell that to the destitute older Black women of East St. Louis!) I mean that the middle generations—the Baby Boomers and the generation after them—have joined in what seems to be a national conspiracy to deny a future to our children.

As our children grow into adulthood, we don't see a need to pass bond issues to support schools. As our kids leave home, we don't feel so strongly about having parks and playgrounds and child services, and we vote accordingly. We become stingy about taxes, complaining about our property assessments, conveniently forgetting that it was other people's property taxes that educated us and our children. Elderly, middle-aged, and young adult alike, we are unwilling to grant to other children what we were given when we were young. And in our zest for tax cuts and deficit spending, we are guaranteeing that they will have less than what earlier voters gave us.

3. Gun control. It is estimated that 55 to 60 percent of American households have at least one gun; many households have entire arsenals. Of course, if you're going to have a handgun, it's because you want to shoot bad guys, so you have to keep the thing loaded and easily available (spare me the National Rifle Association argument about militias and hunting weapons, please; there is no need to keep them loaded). Unfortunately, the odds of your being able to save your family with your little gun are much lower than the odds that one of your children or one of your neighbors' children will blow himself or herself or someone else away with your little gun.

Yes, criminals have guns. They always will, although we could make it a damned sight harder for them to get them by banning the manufacture, importation, sale, possession, and use of many types of weapons, starting with assault weapons and handguns. But if we simply arm everyone in response, we are making the problem worse. And the guns we buy and keep around will kill our children. They will shoot themselves, or we will shoot them (accidentally or on purpose), or they will get shot because they got between two gangs, or they will get shot because they joined a gang—and yes, I do have sympathy for some gang members, especially if they happen to be 10 or 12 years old.

As long as we tolerate the free and easy proliferation of handguns and assault weapons, we are tolerating the murder of our children.

4. Family planning. The issue of abortion rights, with all its complications and delicacies, has been dragged into the political arena, and it will not escape that spotlight any time soon. Too often lost in the debate is the fact that the easiest way to avoid abortion is to avoid unwanted pregnancy.

To me, there is an absolute moral obligation on the part of those who would ban abortion to prevent unwanted pregnancy and to protect every unwanted child who is born. We do neither. We squabble about providing family planning information to teenagers. We fight over providing condoms, despite the skyrocketing number of pediatric and teenaged AIDS patients. We deny decent levels of federal funding for counseling kids about sexual choices. We teach abstinence to hormone-ravaged young people. We pretend that teenaged homosexuals don't exist. And if an unwanted child is born who happens to have deficiencies of one sort or another, we don't want that child, either, and we leave him or her to grow up in an institution.

And so the abortion battle goes on, moving farther and farther away from any pretense of interest in what happens to children, especially pregnant children and their offspring. Yet we know that being born unwanted, or being born to one too young, marks a child as a candidate for abuse.

5. **War.** We like war. We're good at it. We spend a lot of money on it. And sometimes it is necessary; the idea of living under the Third Reich does not appeal to me.

But we must understand the consequences of war for children. How can we tolerate the skeletal faces of starving babies in Somalia, literally dying in the streets while armed toughs enjoy their restaurant meals? How can we accept the wholesale deaths of children in Haiti, whose pitiful economy has been devastated by a military coup and the end of its infant democracy? How can we take pride in the slaughter—by bombs, by combat, by disease—of children in Iraq, be they Iraquis, Kurds, or Shiites?

How can we send our young people off to do these deeds? The late songwriter Phil Ochs once lamented, "It's always the old who lead us to the wars; it's always the young who die." We don't just kill other people's children in our wars; we kill our own. And we maim them. And we hurt their hearts and their brains, so that many who cannot overcome their pain end up on our streets. Vietnam veterans are grossly overrepresented among the troubled homeless. The young people whose names are inscribed on the black marble wall in Washington are not the only American children who died in Vietnam.

Sometimes war is necessary, but it is never glorious. It should never be easy. It should never be used as a means of gaining political popularity. It should never be celebrated as some kind of litmus test of our goodness or our strength as a nation. Using children to kill children is wrong. However legitimated it is by history and custom, it is child abuse on a grand and appalling scale.

How much more thrilling it was to see our young people in uniform fanning out into the devastation in south Florida to provide food, housing, comfort, and hope for the tens of thousands of people who had lost everything. How sweet it was to see the special care they were taking with children. How proud I felt when I saw medical students from the University of Florida going door to door (or what were once doors) in the poorest of neighborhoods, into the migrant worker camps, seeking to provide care to families and especially children. How good it was that among the tons of donations there were boxes of toys, from people who understand that kids need roses as well as bread. My God, we can reach out so lovingly to children when there has been a calamity!

When will we start reaching out to them the rest of the time?

Old and In the Way

January 1993

As we embark on the new year, we are also standing on the edge of the 21st century. When we cross into the new millennium, we will probably be the oldest national population on earth, or will be at least tied for that honor with the Swedes and the Japanese. Average American life expectancy today is a bit more than 75 years; it is anticipated to improve marginally, especially for those over 65 (who can expect to live another 17 years). Already, 31 million people (12.6 percent of the population) are older than 65; 3.1 million are over 85.

The Baby Boomers are turning 40 at the rate of 9,000 a day; they start turning 50 in 1996. Thus, by 2010, one in four Americans will be older than 55. Twenty years later, one in three will be older than 55 and one in five will be older than 65. By the year 2050, 16 million Americans could be older than 85.

This is not a revelation. These trends have been eminently predictable since the Baby Boomers started making their appearance in the late 1940s.

Yet we have been curiously resistant to understanding the implications of the aging of Americans. In healthcare, for example, we have failed to successfully encourage growth in the gerontological medical and nursing specialties; we remain far too attached to institutional models of care for those who could benefit from less restrictive options; Medicare continues to ignore basic medical needs of the elderly, from long-term care to eyeglasses and hearing aids; and

Medicaid, destitute as it is, remains the most common (indeed, almost universal) third-party payer of nursing home costs for the aging, despite the fact that it was never intended to serve that purpose.

And we continue, as a society, to hate and fear old people.

I realize the statement sounds harsh, but I can come to no other conclusion in the face of the mumbling I keep hearing out there: "Americans over 65 have the highest income of any age group" (yes, and also a high poverty rate, second only to that of children, who have an inexcusably high rate). "Americans over 65 exercise more political power than any other group" (yes, they do—because they vote. Did you?). "Americans over 65 get most of the entitlements in this country" (given Social Security and Medicare, this is true, but if it's such a horror, why do Baby Boomers keep expressing fears that there won't be any money left for their Medicare and Social Security payments when their time comes?).

And culturally, of course, through advertising and other means, we continue to devalue aging people—especially aging women, who are portrayed as desexed, unattractive, and unworthy of men's attention. A current soft drink commercial implies that if the two elderly women in the ad would just consume this drink, they will look like model Cindy Crawford, half a century younger than they. Or, if an older woman is held up as a figure of glamour, she tends to be someone along the lines of Dyan Cannon or Lauren Hutton, who are hardly typical of the over-50 set. Indeed, the selling of hair coloring to cover gray, cosmetics to mask aging skin, surgery to remove evidence of age (healthcare providers being the marketeers here), and other activities designed to help older people (mostly women) conceal their age is one of the major industries in the United States.

How Much Care?

Given all this, then, it should probably not come as a surprise that much talk in policy circles these days revolves around how much healthcare older people "deserve," and whether Medicare should be means-tested, and why all those nasty old nursing home residents are being allowed to rip off the young women and children who constitute most of the Medicaid population but who receive only about one-fourth of the benefits.

There has also been frank discussion of whether people of advanced age should receive publicly funded healthcare for conditions like cancer. In his courageous (if, in my opinion, dangerously wrong-headed) book, *Setting Limits* (Simon & Schuster, 1987), Daniel Callahan, director of the Hastings Center, proposed that when a person has lived a full "biographical life," that is, has lived to his or her late 70s or early 80s, then "medical care should no longer be oriented to resisting death."

He suggested that relief of suffering, palliative care for the severely chronically ill, and resistance to the application of advanced medical technologies be the principles on which care of the aging should be based. He added that no aging patient should ever be "abandoned." But in public discussion of his proposal, he conceded that if an elderly patient could pay cash out-of-pocket for medical care, he or she should, of course, be allowed to continue to purchase it. Although I was never in favor of Callahan's idea, he lost me completely when I realized that he was really only proposing refusal of care for the elderly poor who were dependent on public funds.

Well, needless to say, Callahan's proposal was downed in a hail of philosophical and moral bullets. It never got far enough to be shot down for political reasons, which would have happened.

Callahan has continued to address the problem, and in his more recent work has urged Americans—all Americans, not just the aging—to think communally and to be willing to engage in at least minor self-restraint in our gluttonous consumption of healthcare, for the sake of the society as a whole and the needs of others. It has proven a quixotic quest.

It *Sounds* Demeaning

The fact that his idea of restricting care for the elderly was shot down in flames might indicate I am wrong in claiming that we devalue older people. This is not the case. Indeed, I don't think the core issue—the fact that we don't find elderly people handy to have around—was ever touched. To quote from Callahan's 1987 work: "The presumption against resisting death after a natural life span would not in any sense demean those who have lived that long or suggest that their lives are less valuable than those of younger people." Well, if you're going to let them die of treatable disease, you're saying that helping them continue to live is of no use to them or us—a proposition that sure *sounds* demeaning to me.

No, the fact is that many of us, in and out of healthcare, believe that the value of someone who has lived three score or four score years is simply less than that of someone who has lived only a few years, and therefore we need not work as hard to procure any more time for them.

The evidence is everywhere, as recent research findings demonstrate. The older a woman gets, the less likely it is that she will be urged by her physician to have a Pap smear—despite the fact that older women are more likely to develop uterine cancer. Only last year did Medicare decide to cover the cost of mammography, despite the fact that breast cancer is much more common among its beneficiaries than among the female population as a whole. One reason medical students have cited for their aversion to the specialty of general internal medicine is that it usually involves caring for elderly patients.

And physicians often tend to be less aggressive in the diagnosis and care of older patients, even if such care could enhance their longevity or quality of life. As John Rowe, MD, now president of Mount Sinai Medical Center in New York City, wrote in his classic 1985 piece, "Too frequently, clinicians are apt to ascribe a disability or abnormal physical or laboratory finding to 'old age,' when the actual cause is a specific disease process" ("Healthcare of the Elderly," *New England Journal of Medicine*, Vol. 312, No. 13, March 28, 1985).

Complicating the situation is a tendency on the part of the elderly to fail to report even serious health conditions. Rowe notes,

"This apparently self-destructive behavior springs from the notion on the part of older people that advanced age is necessarily accompanied by illness and functional decline and that many symptoms are thus to be expected rather than treated."

While this hits us as odd behavior on the part of patients who have guaranteed coverage (and challenges the belief that the elderly "overuse the healthcare system"), why should we wonder at a lack of self-esteem among older Americans in a society that constantly questions their value and openly discusses whether it is worth the trouble to provide them with healthcare?

One point must be made here. Age is used, and should be used, when appropriate, as a clinical standard. A patient can be too old to be a candidate for a particular treatment, just as a patient can be too young for a treatment. A 90-year-old man with chronic obstructive pulmonary disease is unlikely to survive general anesthesia, regardless of how helpful a surgical procedure might be for him. And although the upper age limit for organ transplants has been raised repeatedly, there is still a point of aging beyond which a patient cannot be expected to survive the procedure. My question is simply whether, if we hear of an 85-year-old receiving a liver transplant, and we disapprove, we are doing so because we find it clinically inappropriate or socially inappropriate.

The Roots of Bias

What are the roots of our bias against age? I think there are several reasons we have come to this pass.

We fear aging and what we presume are its accompanying burdens. It isn't just that being older brings with it a sense of being less attractive, for men and women alike. It also brings physical deterioration, and, if we live long enough, it can bring mental and emotional deterioration. Alzheimer's disease can take its place among the dread diseases of our time, as terrifying as cancer or AIDS—and perhaps more so, for many of us. We fear we may not be able to run marathons, have sex, live independently, or eat spicy food. The fact is that older people do all these things, but because we fear that we might not be able to, we devalue aging—and thus the aged. We are afraid of what they may be telling us about our own future.

Most elderly Americans are women, who are already devalued in society. The demographic facts speak for themselves. The majority of people over 50 are women, and three-quarters of those over 85 are women. Tradition, policy, and law all devalue women in American society, so why should aging women be exempt? It is not a coincidence that the predations of Jack Kevorkian, the retired pathologist who has abetted the suicides of five people as of this writing, have been restricted to women. It may be that sick, aging women are more likely to devalue themselves and wish themselves dead, mirroring the values of the society around them. But one still wonders, as professor George Annas of Boston University has asked, what the reaction would be if Kevorkian extended his activities to include sick, younger men among his victims.

On another front, in their disturbing study of how the courts view "right-to-die" cases, Steven Miles, MD, and Allison August concluded that when the patient in question is a man, the patient's rights tend to predominate and be honored in the court decision. When the patient is a woman, the interests of others, including caregivers, family, and even the state, supersede those of the patient. In one case, a retired woman hospital administrator's often-repeated remarks about not wanting to be subjected to life-prolonging technology were rejected by the court after she was disabled by a stroke. The judge reasoned that although she had said these things to many people over a period of years, they were really just emotional reactions to deaths she had witnessed, and could not be taken seriously ("Courts, Gender, and the 'Right to Die'," *Law, Medicine, and Healthcare*, Vol. 18, Nos. 1-2, Spring/Summer 1990).

I think we must face the likelihood that our ignoring of key issues involving the health of the elderly—long-term care and its financing, targeted prevention and health promotion, patients' rights to determine treatment options, and appropriate levels of care—is probably based on the fact that this is a largely female population, not just an aging one.

Past and Future

We hold the future in greater esteem than the past. Ours is a short-term society, ranging from the stupidity of our financial and investment markets and their immediate-return philosophy to the fact that we continually forget our own history. The watchword is "What have you done for me lately?"

This is probably not restricted to Americans; one of the most powerful expressions of this attitude ever seen was when, after Winston Churchill had led Britain and her allies through a horrible war and achieved victory against long odds, the people of England promptly voted him out of office.

We value the promise more than the deed done, the life not yet lived more than the life nearly completed.

Some of this is rooted in religious belief and the common presumption that the new life is innocent and without stain, while those who have been around for a while are doomed to purgatory at best. Some of it is rooted in the tension between what we already know and what we want to learn.

But some of it is rooted in a culturally specific disdain for the knowledge, wisdom, and experience of age. We would rather be young and dumb again, because we want the chance to go back and recoup the wasted time, undo the destructive acts, make right the wrongs. And we can't. So we pin our hopes on our children and others who are younger, hoping they will redeem us—and unconsciously consign those who are older to the ranks of the unredeemable.

Understand that this is not how all people confront aging. Some years ago, philosopher John Kilner went to Africa and worked with the healers of the Akamba people, seeking to find out how they would choose whom to treat if there were only one dose of medicine—the young patient or the older?

He found that "where only one person can be saved, many Akamba favor saving an old man before a young, even where the young man is first in line. . . . Life, they insist, is more than atomistic sums of individual economic contributions; it is a social fabric of interpersonal relations. The older a person becomes, the more intricately interwoven he or she becomes in the lives of others, and the greater the damage done if that person is removed. At the same time, the older person has wisdom—a perspective on life that comes only with age—which is considered to be a particularly important social resource" ("Who Shall Be Saved? An African Answer," Hastings Center Report, Vol. 14, No. 3, June 1984).

Many Akamba also believe that if there is only one dose of medicine, it should be divided among the two patients, even if that lessens or even cancels its effectiveness. This, you see, would be fair, even if not cost-effective by our definition.

Until we can learn to honor what people have done in the past, and build that into the equation of what they are worth to us when they are perhaps frail, or cantankerous, or demented, the Akamba will be way ahead of us.

Forever Young

There is in a collection of Ray Bradbury stories called *The October Country* a tale of a man who, when he was a boy, lost his young girlfriend through drowning when they were swimming. Decades later, swimming at the same beach, he mysteriously encounters her corpse, still young and beautiful. He muses that she will always be young and beautiful, and that he will love her forever. There were people in my life who are also frozen in their youth through death: David, dead at 27; Stan, dead at 33; Marsha, dead at 34; Steve, dead at 36. They will always be young and beautiful, and they will always be my friends.

But that will not be the case for most of us, nor has that been the case with those who are today in their 60s, 70s, 80s, and beyond. It is not simply the fact that if we set up policies that vilify and punish the elderly of today, those policies will vilify and punish us when we are the elderly of tomorrow. Nor is it a matter of ignoring crucial policy questions, such as Social Security payments and Medicare coverage for millionaires, the time bomb of long-term care, overtreating older patients simply because they have Medicare and supplemental coverage, or undertreating them after luring them into managed care programs that inappropriately leverage access to care. These are real issues that must be solved.

It is simply my hope that, as we address these extraordinarily painful questions, we will do so with a sensitivity to and respect for our older brethren as enriching factors in our society, not as used-up inconveniences who are not worth our time. For our time is their time; they bought it for us, and we should protect it for them.

Above the Law

March 1993

Maybe it was Michael Milken's sentence being reduced. Maybe it was Woody Allen's interview on "60 Minutes," in which I got the impression that he just didn't think the rules applied to him. Maybe it was the Keating Five getting a slap on the wrist from the Senate after enabling the predation of one of the worst savings and loan sharks.

Maybe it was earlier, when I watched Fawn Hall (Oliver North's secretary, remember?) testifying before Congress that she violated the United States Constitution because she thought she was obeying a higher law. Then there was US Attorney General Edwin Meese—the highest-ranking law enforcement official in the nation—suavely assuring a press conference that because he had not been indicted, he obviously was innocent. That led to my coining the Ed Meese Rule: If you didn't get caught, you didn't do it.

I don't know which of these events was the spark. But I have been thinking about the notion of being above the law, about the fact that quite a few of us seem convinced that the rules don't apply where we're concerned. Healthcare folk are particularly susceptible to this.

Of course, we don't admit to it. A suggestion that we think we're beyond the reach of the rules will be met with a pious and almost automatic response that "no one should be above the law." But the fact is that we all jaywalk, we all park illegally now and again, we all try to zip in and out of the dry cleaner's without putting the quarter in the parking meter, we all drive a few miles an hour above the limit—and, sooner or later, most of us get caught.

And when we get caught, we resent it. Even if we know we have been caught fair and square, we somehow feel that a wrong has been done to us, that we don't deserve our fate.

This is extremely human, and usually it does little harm except to the integrity of our own moral beliefs about crime and punishment. In most cases, the sin is one of hypocrisy. It's only when we graduate to talking bankers into using people's pension funds to buy worthless junk bonds, or when we try to get away with murder or brutalizing the Constitution, that our violation of the rules becomes a social crime with actual or potentially devastating consequences.

Why Do We Do It?

But why, when we know it's wrong to violate the accepted laws and rules of our society, do we do it anyway?

In the first place, I think we are just more willing to accept limits that apply to someone else and not to us. When we're standing in line at the Post Office, and someone is taking half an hour with some complicated transaction and filling out forms at the counter that should have been filled out ahead of time, we get angry. But when we are at the counter and realize that we didn't fill out the forms, then that's just an honest mistake and the people standing in line behind us should be more understanding.

In healthcare, it's that other hospital that's trying to bamboozle the planning agency into approving a certificate of need for an utterly unnecessary new wing; when it's my hospital, I know my community will be well served by that wing, even if our occupancy rate currently is only 23 percent. It's just a temporary slump.

And, of course, all the unnecessary cesareans are done at that other place; all of ours are justified. There may be voices whispering that we are lying to ourselves, but as songwriter Paul Simon wrote, "A man hears what he wants to hear and disregards the rest."

Another reason for our hypocrisy is that we don't realize it's hypocrisy. We really believe that our behavior is so exemplary that there is no need to regulate it. In fact, we resent the implication that there is a need for social oversight of our activities.

One of the most common expressions of this, of course, is the argument that "if guns are outlawed, only outlaws will have guns," based on the (erroneous) assumption that everyone else who owns a gun acquires, stores, and uses it in the most responsible possible way. Thus there is no reason, those who hold this belief say, to regulate or ban any weapon. It simply never enters their heads that a non-outlaw drunk with an assault weapon or an untrained hunter running around a populated area with a loaded rifle is every bit as dangerous as a habitual criminal with a handgun.

In healthcare, of course, which certainly has its share of regulation, there is a general resentment of many of those strictures. Of course we dispose of toxic waste responsibly. Of course we scrutinize applicants for clinical privileges carefully. Of course we respect the confidentiality of patient medical records. We wouldn't think of doing anything less; why don't you trust us? We believe there is no need to tell us to do the right thing, or to threaten us with penalties if we don't, because we always do the right thing.

The problem, of course, is that toxic hospital waste has appeared on beaches, unlicensed physicians have wreaked damage on patients because their credentials weren't sufficiently checked by hospital authorities, and patient medical records have become the subject of inhouse gossip and have been leaked to insurers, the press, and others.

Rules and laws are not there to protect us from those who are pure of heart and scrupulous of behavior; they are there to protect us from those who are less well intentioned or are just plain sloppy. We should not be so resentful or feel that we are not being trusted. As someone once said, surprise inspections shouldn't frighten people who are doing a good job. (They do, anyway, of course, just as a notice of audit from the Internal Revenue Service will send even the most honest taxpayer into cardiac arrest. We'll discuss that another time.)

The "Yes, But . . ." Defense

Most of us, at some point in our personal or professional lives, find ourselves in a situation in which we are well aware of the presence of rules or laws, and are well aware that they apply to us. And we respect these constraints and their intent; we just think we are exceptions. We think we have a valid reason for breaking the rules. Certainly that was what Fawn Hall had in mind. Certainly that was what Oliver North had in mind. And that was what Nazi strategist Joseph Goebbels had in mind when he said that to be able to slaughter Jews and Gypsies and still remain "decent men" was what made the Nazis "great."

This is the "yes, but . . ." defense of violation of community standards, rules, or laws: Yes, I know this limit is here, and here for a good reason, but I'm the exception.

Healthcare, of course, often sees itself as an exception. And there are rules to which healthcare *is* an exception. Despite insistence to the contrary by market-oriented academic economists (many of whom have never even witnessed, let alone been involved in, the processes of patient care), healthcare does not obey the rules of marketplace economics, and it never will. Healthcare is neither purely a business nor purely a human service, and no amount of posturing will change that.

But by the same coin, healthcare's belief that it is inherently morally superior is ill-founded. Responsible healthcare is moral; irresponsible healthcare is not. We generally see Mother Teresa as a moral representative of religion; we generally do not see Jim Bakker in that same light.

And although the board members and administrators of each hospital believe their institution is special, that its mission is more keenly felt, that it is more needed than others, that it deserves special treatment because it is 100 years old or has a teaching mission or whatever, that position is only rarely justified. Indeed, it is amazing how many institutions have been able to make that case, so that we currently have special treatment of (among others) isolated rural hospitals, rural referral centers, teaching hospitals, children's hospitals, financially distressed hospitals, and several other kinds of hospitals. One sometimes wonders if there are hospitals that are *not* exceptions!

A Downward Spiral

No matter how deeply held is the belief that one is above the law, or that one should be exempted from a law that applies to everyone else, there are two major problems with this position, aside from niceties like moral honesty. The first is that if even a few members of a society decide they are above the law, then soon there is no law.

For example, we have seen time and time again that someone must take the lead in order for looting to start. That was Spike Lee's point in the scene in *Do the Right Thing* when the protagonist, surrounded by people waiting for something to happen, throws the garbage can into the pizza parlor and starts the riot; the look on his face is that of a man who knows *someone* is going to put a match to the fire, so he might as well do it and get it over with.

And once the rules are declared irrelevant, a downward spiral results, whether it is in south central Los Angeles, Bosnia-Herzegovina, or Somalia. If the rules are ignored by some, they will be ignored by more and more, and ultimately there are no rules.

Although healthcare, fortunately, has shown more self-discipline than the lawless toughs of Somalia, we have created situations such as a town of 30,000 people with five MRI machines, a nine-hospital county with nine open-heart surgery programs, and entire sections of states where no physician will accept a Medicaid patient.

Recently a 38-year-old man died of septicemia in Hawaii because he was a Medicaid beneficiary and could find no oral surgeon to treat his abscessed tooth. If providers do not have to accept Medicaid patients, the situation can and does arise in which none of them will. (This is not meant to be an argument that providers should be forced to accept Medicaid patients, but it does illustrate that the absence of such a requirement can leave patients with no options.)

The second problem with believing that we are above the law is that when we do so arrogantly or without just cause, we make it harder for those around us to decide when exceptions should, in fact, be made. For the fact is that there are very few laws—if any—that are so perfect that no exceptions to them should be allowed.

There is a rich ethics literature on this, as well as complex and troubling human history. Take "Thou shalt not kill," for example, which is often viewed as one of the more absolute moral laws of society. All one need do to shake us up on this one is to ask if, knowing what we know today, you had the chance to kill Hitler before he came to power—even if he were unarmed and defenseless—would you do it? And if there were no exceptions to "Thou shalt not steal," no nation would be able to run effective intelligence operations.

Human beings have faced terrible dilemmas on this score. After an explosion destroyed much of Halifax, Nova Scotia in 1917, many people were hopelessly buried in debris that began to burn. A rescuer who had tried to save them later said his deepest regret was that he had not brought his gun with him, in order to kill them and save them the pain of dying by fire.

And, of course, one of the key issues in the Nuremberg trials of German war criminals was the question of whether one could be excused for committing atrocities because one was a sworn member of the military and had been ordered to commit atrocities. The Nuremberg tribunal's decision was uncompromising: "I was just following orders" is not an acceptable excuse for violating rules of human decency.

So one of the worst reasons for frivolously claiming that one has a right to be exempted from rules others are expected to follow is that it weakens the case for exemption when it should occur. For this reason, I believe that, in or out of healthcare, we should be very careful about thinking the rules don't apply to us.

A Few Parameters

But what do you do when you really think you must violate a rule or law or other social constraint?

This, too, is a tangled area of ethics, especially in healthcare. One of the great essays in this regard is "Who Should Live When Not All Can Live?" by James Childress, which was published in *Soundings* in 1969 and is also reprinted in my first ethics book (*Making Choices*, American Hospital Publishing, 1986). His basic point is that there is always a need for exceptions to tough rules, but those exceptions must be rare, must be very difficult to obtain, must be granted to prevent harm rather than to achieve benefit, and must be to the advantage of the general community, not just one individual. (One of his examples is that even if a particular medical procedure is not available, an exception should be made for the president of the United States if our nation is at war and its survival has been threatened.)

In keeping with that philosophy, I suggest that if you really think you must break a rule or law, you should seek an exception, rather than just ignoring or violating the constraint and hoping you won't get caught. After all, if your cause is just, you run a good chance of succeeding.

So the issue is whether your reason is good enough. And to that end, I want to recommend a few parameters for judging whether what you want to do justifies breaking the rules. These standards, I hope, can be applied by both individuals and organizations.

1. What is the rule or law in question? There is a difference between parking illegally and walking into a cafeteria firing a submachine gun. There is a difference between using the emergency department photocopier for a personal project and refusing to treat a patient with a ruptured aorta because you just did your nails. Social constraints such as codes, regulations, and laws vary in seriousness, and violating some is much more serious than violating others.

The test is, as a rule, the effect on other human beings (or other living things), either individually or in the broader sense of the community or society. The hierarchy tends to run from rules whose violation harms no one to rules whose violation causes death or great suffering; generally, the more people who suffer, the more grave the violation. But yes, we have different rules for war and for the poor, unfortunately.

2. What is the goal of the rule or law? Again, there are degrees of seriousness attached to various constraints, based on what they are intended to do. Parking meters are as much a source of revenue as they are a source of social benefit; parking too long at a meter might rob another motorist of a chance to use the space, but the city treasury benefits from the expired meter. On the other hand, we have rules against the sloppy disposal of medical materials contaminated with HIV for a much more serious reason. So it is not just the subject a rule addresses; it is the *reason* the rule exists.

3. What are the consequences of breaking the rule or law? If you park too long at a meter, you've been selfish, but that's hardly the same thing as parking in a space reserved for disabled drivers or in a space next to a fire hydrant. There's a wonderful little moral essay in the otherwise morally muddled film *Backdraft*, in which the firefighters, without a moment's hesitation, smash the front windows of a car parked at a fire hydrant and run the hose through the front seat of the car. It's a great illustration of the differential consequences of breaking rules: The driver parked at the hydrant and, as a consequence, no longer has front windows. The firemen smashed his windows in pursuit of a higher cause. It is very unlikely that they would be punished for their actions.

But if that driver had parked at the hydrant in order to rush a choking baby into an emergency room, then she was justified in taking the risk of blocking the hydrant for a short time. Her parking at the hydrant because she did not want to walk a block from a legal parking space would not be viewed so benignly.

One of our problems in healthcare is that we seem to have trouble understanding the consequences of our actions. Whenever a highly publicized incidence of malpractice occurs, most of us wonder how the people involved could not have seen what would inevitably happen as the result of what they did. Yet we insulate ourselves from the consequences of our own actions. In doing so, we make it easier to trivialize rules that are supposed to govern our behavior.

4. Should I just go ahead and break the rule or should I seek an exemption? There are times when just breaking the rule is the best approach, such as refusing an order to send people to the gas chamber or smashing car windows in order to stop a fire. Most of the time, however, I think seeking an exemption is better. It makes us more accountable than does trying to sneak around the constraint, which in turn leads us to consider much more carefully whether our rule breaking is worth it. It brings other people into the decisionmaking process, which is usually a good idea, in that we are likely to make less selfish decisions.

Besides, having others watching us creates what is known in research as the Hawthorne effect—the fact that we behave differently when we know we are being watched. And we generally behave better.

Also, seeking an exemption shows respect for the rule or law and, although it weakens it in some ways, it is far less destructive than blatant ignoring of the law. And in my opinion, openly and honestly seeking an exemption often strengthens the rule, because it helps keep it flexible and compassionate. That's why we give judges and juries a good deal of leeway in the sentencing of criminals, and why, even in capital cases, the possibility of pardon, commutation, or clemency is there until the last.

The Oldest Democracy

We are a nation of mavericks, dedicated to individual liberty, and none of us likes to confront the specter of constraint. As one of my students at Boston University, Donald Statuto, MD, observed about rationing, it conjures up the image that Americans are like everyone else and are subject to the same natural limits. That is not something to which we submit willingly. On the other hand, there is a reason that we are the oldest continuing democracy on earth, and that once again, we are witnessing a peaceful, orderly transfer of presidential power at a time when the ability of the Russians or the Haitians to do the same is in grave doubt. The judge was right when he said ours is a government of laws and not of men. Healthcare is no different.

Thus, despite our individualism, our belief in our own moral superiority, and our conviction that we do not need to be monitored or scolded, we should keep in mind Bob Dylan's admonition about those who claim to be special: "If you live outside the law, you must be honest."

Concepts of Community

May 1993

When we speak of communities in the context of serving them as healthcare providers, we tend to think of either the people in our service area (however we define that) or a subset of people in our service area (such as those who have insurance or who belong to the HMO with which we are affiliated). Or else we think of birds of similar feather to our own (such as "the not-for-profit hospital community"). But these are only three types of communities. And often healthcare folk misdirect their mission by not understanding the many concepts of community that are woven into their lives.

So I think it is important to ask: What is a community? What are these clumps we form with each other?

The First Loyalty

For eons, the community of location was the community of first loyalty, because for a very long time, the world was rural. It didn't have many people in it (especially after the bubonic plague wiped out 25 percent of Europe during the 14th century), and we hadn't invented subways yet. The local community was one's world. And it was, of necessity, a communal environment. People shared, whether or not they wanted to, because they had to. And one identified with the place where one was born, lived, and would probably die.

The coming of transportation changed all that. In his brilliant book about change, *Connections*, James Burke describes the results in Great Britain of the coming of the railroads: Towns in which everyone had been a blue-eyed redhead for years suddenly started sprouting brunettes; mining towns where everyone was five feet tall started developing tall children. The isolated gene pools in all those rural areas started to mix, because people discovered that you were not doomed from birth to marry the girl or boy next door. Mobility shattered the insularity of the community of location.

But even in a society of nomads, where we move around with the ease of the Bedouin, our sense of community of location has not left us. People from Chicago, even if they are glad they are from Chicago as opposed to still living there, retain a strong affection for the place, and continue to follow the antics of the Cubs and the Bears decades after they themselves have fled to warmer climes.

I was recently at a dinner party populated by ex-New Yorkers, many of whom did not know each other. During a conversation about New York City street games, I committed the unpardonable sin of mentioning "porch ball." I was hooted down by those at the table, who explained that it's stoop ball, not porch ball ("People in *Boston* play porch ball, Emily"). The waitress was also a former resident of the Big Apple, and she agreed about the proper name of the game.

We still are bound together by the first real estate we trod.

Each of us might still hold membership in a particular community of location, frozen in time, because that community would be its unique old self whenever we went back to it. But once radio and television invaded the hometown, the notion of community of location changed forever. These media started the homogenization process, and much community uniqueness disappeared. Nowhere was this illustrated better than in a recent national news broadcast from Somalia, where a young Somali man, realizing he was being filmed, broke into a faithful version of Michael Jackson's "moonwalk."

Over time, the isolated community with which we identified began to resemble other communities, and soon they all had McDonald's and Holiday Inns and blackened redfish, and, as a result, the link of identification with a single community weakened in us.

This is an inevitable process, and it has its good side. With travel and TV, people started to come into contact with people who were not like themselves. Communications media and the concrete ribbons draped across the land brought black people into contact with white folks, northerner with southerner, Pole with Polynesian. We may not have exactly clasped each other to our bosoms, but we became more aware of who was out there.

Today the community of location is not dead, just weakened. People still feel an acute loyalty to the places where they spent their early years, even if those places are more like each other than they had been. And we still always share something with someone from home. If you're from Brooklyn, you're from Brooklyn; you will never really be from anywhere else.

But the community of location has been and is being augmented by other communities, because human beings can no more live without community than they can live without air. They need to band together, and they do so with the tenacity of Krazy Glue. So as communities of location weaken, others become stronger.

The Shared Event

Today, we also belong to communities of experience: groups of people who have undergone a common event. One example is people who went to the same school. This is a powerful bond, if it can be judged by the amount of money alumni spend on their alma maters.

These communities can be critical, professionally. For example, in some firms, you can be hired simply because you went to Dartmouth Business School. Likewise, there are places where you could never get a job because you went to Dartmouth Business School.

Cross-generational, lasting networks develop, based on the shared experience of being a Yalie or a Duke Blue Devil or a Berkeley Golden Bear. It doesn't matter that my experiences at Berkeley in the mid-Sixties had about as much in common with the experiences of a member of the Cal class of 1928 as scuba diving has with baking brioche; the shared experience is still a bond.

The community of experience allows people who didn't know they had a link to each other to connect. For example, how many people have been joined in a sense of community by what they have seen on television? Think of the comfort TV provided in the days after the killing of John Kennedy, or the enormous impact that the "Roots" series had on our understanding of each other.

Another example, and one of my favorites, is the community of Americans who have been to China. Whether at conferences, on airplanes, in taxis, or elsewhere, I always have something to talk about with someone who has been to China. Travel there is so difficult and the experience of Chinese history and society so overwhelming that everyone I have ever met who has been through it wants to talk about it.

On the other hand, if the shared experience is negative, it can breed poisonous beliefs. It is common, for example, for people who have experienced something unpleasant from a member of a different ethnic group to hate and fear members of that group.

United Against Tigers

What can develop then is a community of fear: people who are drawn together because of their fear of something or someone. It is probably the oldest and most unfortunate form of community, likely born back when people came together because sabre-toothed tigers were on the prowl. Fear, in fact, may have been why people first formed stable social groups beyond the family.

What is positive about communities of fear is the fact that most of us are united against copperheads, certain wild mushrooms, black widow spiders, and forest fires. I would hate to think that these things would become the focus of a community of experience, rather than of a community of fear.

The frightening aspects of this form of community are known to all of us. Fear feeds on itself, and although it can draw people together, that is not always a healthy bond.

But whenever a community of fear forms, we should remember the warnings of writers Gerald Weissman, MD, and Toni Morrison about fearing "the other." Human beings have a love-hate relationship with that which is different. If a woman speaks Tamil or a man wears what we perceive to be a skirt, we are wary. The same society that casts longing eyes at the universe in the hope that someone else is out there does not trust members of its own species who look or act different. And where distrust lurks, there blooms the community of fear.

Into the Same Thing

Another form of community is the community of interest: groups of people who are into the same thing—backgammon, football, French cooking, the stock market, sailing, whatever. We hang out with people who like to do the same things we like to do. We seek people who think like we do. A community of interest gives us something common to talk about and also provides us with opportunities to meet and connect with other people.

What is negative about communities of interest, of course, is that the people who join them can have a bad case of tunnel vision, and they can become exclusionary rather than inclusionary. Interesting as I might find a group of joggers for a few hours, a steady diet of conversation focusing on the relative merits of Nike and Reebok running shoes soon takes on the same thrill as watching paint dry. Furthermore, the focus of the community is so narrow that its members can spend their lives discussing one tiny topic while Rome burns.

Nevertheless, the community of interest may become the dominant form of community in this global village. There is both hope and danger in that thought. The hope is that in a good community of interest, anyone can play.

Watch fiddlers or chess players sometime: Old, young, brown, white, southern, French-Canadian, English-speaking, German-speaking—it doesn't matter. When they share the fiddle, or chess, other differences are forgotten. That's the true hope of the Olympic Games—politics, cheating, boycotts, and terrorists notwithstanding. Shared interests create democracy wherever they are found.

The danger is that those who do not share the interest are forgotten. Those of us who belong to communities of interest—and we all do—need to keep in mind that whatever our subject of interest, fewer people share it than do not share it.

Keeping the Faith

Sometimes a community is formed around something we believe: a community of values. Religious communities (formal and informal), for example, represent people who have come together because they share a sense of spirituality and order that is meaningful to them. These are communities of faith.

But these communities can confuse faith with absolute truth. To me, the glory of faith is that it exists in the absence of scientific proof that it is correct. Unfortunately, sometimes we assume that our faith represents absolute truth, that our religion or our ideology is the only right one. That not only makes us insensitive; it can lead to chauvinism, bigotry, war, and death. In these hair-trigger days, it is ever so easy to cross the thin line between values and prejudice.

Even aside from a blind conviction about the rightness of the cause, communities of values can still be very harsh. Take our standards of beauty, which are impossible for most people to meet. More important, take our standards for what constitute "acceptable" looks, a value that is shallow and destructive.

I was at my local drugstore a couple of years ago, and as I left, I noticed a man standing in the shadow of the door. His nose was horribly mutilated, either by disease or accident. It didn't look like a nose; it looked like something that did not belong on a human face. Before I could stop myself, I looked away.

I was reminded then of something written in the Fifties by a veteran whose face had been shattered by a bullet during the Korean War. He had undergone dozens of operations at a time when reconstructive surgery was of only marginal help, as surgeons strove to give him something resembling socially "acceptable" looks. "Your face," he wrote, "is your passport to the world." It is a passport many of us are too willing to revoke. As members of communities of value, we should take care to avoid those values that, although widely accepted, are only skin deep.

The best way to combat chauvinism, prejudice, shallowness, and the other pitfalls of communities of values is to remember that there are other such communities whose values do not agree with yours. My favorite story about this concerns the Johns Hopkins Hospital in Baltimore. (I am told the story is true, but it may be apocryphal.) Decades ago, a generous donor gave the hospital a lovely statue of Jesus Christ that stands in a sunlit atrium in the rotunda dome of the hospital's most historic building.

One day a Hopkins executive was conducting a tour for prestigious visitors from Asia. They had seen all the high-technology wonders of the hospital, but the executive had saved the building with the classic rotunda and statue for last.

The group came around the corner into the atrium, and the guide paused to allow them to drink in the beautiful sight before he told them the history of the statue. During this pause, one of the awestruck visitors turned to the executive, pointed to the statue, and said, with wonder, "And this—this must be Johns Hopkins!"

The Bonds of Time

Then there are communities of age. The great example is teenagers, who, no matter when they were born, live in a world they purposely create to exclude the rest of us. Another, more powerful community of age is the baby boomers, that great glob of 76 million people born between 1946 and 1964. Boomers think everyone is their age, and it is true that one of every three Americans falls into this age group. They tend to forget that two out of three Americans do not.

A community of time is similar to a community of age, except that its members are united by having been around at a certain time. People who lived through the Depression, World War II, or the Sixties belong to specific communities of time. These communities are delicate, but they can embody the best of the human spirit (see "A Community of Time").

Central to Them All

These are some of the communities to which we belong.

In his somewhat depressing portrait of an America losing its sense of communality, *Habits of the Heart,* philosopher Robert Bellah writes of a man who describes his Shangri-La as being a castle with a moat; he would like to take those he cares about inside the castle and just pull up the drawbridge and shut the world out. But even as we become more and more of an enclave society, look around: Whether they involve locality, experience, interest, fear, values, age, or time, communities are forming and dissolving, taking the place of traditional communities, and developing into the places and people who will be the focus of healthcare service in the 21st century.

For healthcare is central to all these communities. In its most limited sense, the community of location served by a provider organization—whether it is a small town in North Dakota or the constituencies of the sprawling Kaiser-Permanente empire—is dependent upon that provider for its care in its hour of need. In the larger sense, we are all members of a community of experience that involves having been ill or injured or caring about someone who has. That is one of the largest, most fragile, and most universal communities on earth.

Healthcare's communities of fear are many, but those of greatest concern are providers who fear change, who fear "the other" (whoever that is), or who fear other providers, for these fears block progress, collaboration, and justice. They also make us insensitive to the basic healthcare community of fear, which is the shared unease, fright, or terror of patients and families who do not know what the outcome of their healthcare experience will be. It is their fears we need to allay, even at the price of our own.

There are also many communities of interest in healthcare, more than can be mentioned here. But three to which I hope we all belong are the communities devoted to improving the health of *all* those around us, to achieving access to care for all, and to providing our services at a price that society can afford.

These interests are, of course, expressions of the deeper community of values that states that healing, justice, and equity must guide what we believe and do. If we commit ourselves to those values, we can continue our progress toward creating a healthcare community that will stand—ever-changing, but always present—for all ages and all time.

. . . .

A Community of Time

In many rural English villages, the carnage of World War I slaughtered an entire generation of young English manhood—along with the young men of France, Germany, Australia, Austria, and other places—in the interest of preserving crumbling imperial societies.

Traditionally, in rural England, on certain holidays, a form of ritual dance called "morris dancing" took place, in which only the village men were allowed to participate. It involves wearing bells and ribbons and doing very athletic, sometimes almost violent dance steps. It's quite pagan and is carried on to this day by dedicated dancers in both North America and Great Britain, who constitute one of the most charming, and obsessive, communities of interest you will find anywhere.

But it almost didn't turn out that way, for many of the men didn't come back from World War I. The dances, which were specific to each village, could have been doomed. But they did not die because the women in some hamlets, faced with breaking a taboo or losing a tradition, picked up the bells, the ribbons, the swords, and the garlands, and danced the morris themselves in order to save it.

English poet Austin John Marshall wrote a poem about these women, "Dancing at Whitsun," which goes, in part:

It's fifty long springtimes since she was a bride,
But still you may see her at each Whitsuntide,
In a dress of white linen with ribbons of green,
As green as her memories of loving.

The feet that were nimble tread carefully now,
As gentle a measure as age will allow,
Through groves of white blossoms, by fields of young corn,
Where once she was pledged to her true love.

Down from the green farmlands and from their loved ones,
Marched husbands and brothers and fathers and sons,
There's a fine roll of honor where the Maypole once stood,
And the ladies go dancing at Whitsun.

There's a straight row of houses in these latter days
All covering the downs where the sheep used to graze,
There's a field of red poppies—a gift from the Queen—
And the ladies go dancing at Whitsun.

Managed Care and Managing Ethics

July 1993

Three things I need to make clear right off the bat: First, when I speak (or write) of managed care, I do not mean "managed competition" (or whatever the Jackson Hole Group/Stanford business school/Clinton Administration healthcare reform idea is calling itself these days). I mean the use of capitated payment, health maintenance organizations or other forms of integrated care, and primary care "gatekeeping."

Second, I am a big fan of appropriate, quality-minded, ethically operated managed care. I have belonged to HMOs much of my life and am a former employee of the Kaiser Foundation Health Plan. I am particularly impressed by not-for-profit staff or group model HMOs in which most or all individual and institutional providers belong to the same organization.

Third, managed care, in and of itself, is a neutral notion. It can be done well or poorly, and the motivation behind it can range from a desire to provide coordinated, comprehensive, high-quality care to a desire to reap vast profits by denying proper access to sick people who can't fight back or don't know they are being victimized. We have seen ample evidence of both over the years.

That having been said, there are ethics issues specific to managed care, and, as the healthcare reform debate rambles (or stumbles) on, some of those issues deserve a closer look.

Some ethics concerns voiced in connection with managed care, of course, are ideological in nature and have more to do with physicians' or other providers' preferred practice settings than they do with patient-centered ethics questions.

For example, it is often stated that a physician who is on salary or a tight contract cannot possibly put the patient's interests first. This implies that a physician in fee-for-service, independent practice automatically puts the patient's interest first. Both ideas are absurd; selfishness, greed, and honor are not determined by the structure of a physician's practice.

It is also often said that managed care, because it encourages (or even requires) a more conservative pattern of care than is seen in unbridled fee-for-service practice, automatically means rationing and skimping on care. Well, conservative care does often mean "rationing," in that it tends to be less lavish in its use of some healthcare resources, such as inpatient hospitalization and some forms of tertiary care. But that is not the same as skimping or denying useful services. Furthermore, we have all seen the kind of damage that can be done by overzealous care, overuse of tests, unnecessary surgery, and endless prolongation of existence with no benefit to patients; it certainly belies the argument that uncontrolled use of health services is a superior model.

Issues of turf, control, and who gets the money are, by and large, ideological and political and should not be confused with some of the deeper ethics questions that managed care presents. Here are a few of those deeper questions:

Are the incentives for providers in managed care arrangements any more "perverse" than the incentives in fee-for-service care? Some people believe that healthcare providers (especially physicians, who are a popular target just now) are motivated only by money, and that how they are paid determines how they practice. Others say that as professionals, providers are singularly resistant to issues of payment. The reality lies in the vast ground between those two positions.

We must concede that physicians and hospitals, to a degree, are influenced by payment incentives. If there is more money to be made in doing more, there is certainly at least a temptation, if not a tendency, to do more. In the case of for-profit activity, in fact, not to do more would be a violation of one's fiduciary responsibility to one's stockholders. (That's why I am so suspicious about healthcare for-profits, but that's another column.) Fee-for-service care, then, is often described as giving "perverse" incentives to providers.

Managed care turns traditional incentives on their heads in two ways. First, it makes conservative care the standard and tries to promote conservative use of resources as a culture within the organization. Second, it commonly relies on capitation—a lump sum paid for the care of each patient, pretty much regardless of diagnosis. Thus to do more reduces profit, rather than enhancing it. This incentive, too, has the possibility of being "perverse."

The question is how the ethical provider reduces the possibility of being unduly or inappropriately influenced by the fiscal consequences of his or her actions. This, to me, is the real question, and it applies across all of healthcare, managed or not.

The answer, not surprisingly, is to define ethical and professional standards that are appropriate—putting the patient's interest first, using clinical and scientific rather than financial criteria in making patient care decisions, adhering to accepted standards of quality, and using outcomes data—and to behave in accordance with those standards.

But that really is not enough. In accepting the mantle of professionalism and the high degree of freedom that it allows (and, despite all the carping, healthcare professionals do have much more freedom than people in most other lines of work), one also accepts the responsibility to speak out and to resist when unethical practices are being pursued. That includes unacceptable behavior on the part of peers and unacceptable demands by payers, regulators, or the organization with which one is affiliated.

Nor is it sufficient to say, "This outfit is asking me to do unethical things," and quit. That protects the provider, but it does nothing to protect current and future patients. One must do what one can to see that the unethical practices are ended. Sadly, healthcare professionals have a pretty bleak record when it comes to turning their colleagues in or speaking out against organizations that provide poor care.

This brotherhood (and sisterhood) of silence has led to some terrible things, such as the scandalous Florida HMO, International Medical Centers, with its poor care and organized crime connections, and the forcing of Medicaid mothers and children into dubious managed care arrangements that clamp down inappropriately on their access while at the same time denying them what had been the "safety net" of the emergency room.

In all probability, this concern will become more vexing in coming years. If there is more money to be made in denying care than in overproviding it, rest assured that the profiteers, the entrepreneurs, the fast-buck artists, and the marginal providers will flood into managed care the way they once flooded into fee-for-service quackery. As James Bentley, vice president of the American Hospital Association, has pointed out, if we aren't careful, the brokers of care could end up being three guys on the second floor of the bank building, smoking cigars and cutting discount deals with providers. And if healthcare professionals remain silent about such things, or voice concerns only about their own situation and not about risks to patients, sleaziness will prevail.

Should patients be denied the right to choose their own physician? This is another accusation leveled consistently at managed care: that one is assigned a physician, or must choose from a limited list of physicians, or cannot count on having the same physician all the way through a course of treatment or a pregnancy.

The argument can be well founded; most managed care arrangements, one way or another, limit choice of physician. However, these days, so does almost every other arrangement. Preferred provider arrangements, which are not managed care but, rather, discount deals, limit choice of provider unless the patient is willing to pay more to go to a nonpreferred physician. "Exclusive provider" arrangements can direct patients to a small selection of doctors, perhaps only those in one group practice or on one hospital's medical staff.

And what kind of freedom of choice of hospital do most patients have these days? The 1992 KPMG Peat Marwick study of employee health benefits found that 96 percent of individuals covered by employer-sponsored plans now have limitations of some kind on their ability to seek care and/or choose providers. So free choice of provider has become something of a myth, except for the Medicare population.

Even if such freedom still existed, I think it is fair to say that patients and prospective patients rarely choose physicians on the basis of hard outcomes data, demonstrated quality, or other objective criteria. Usually, we choose on the basis of the "real estate rule" (location, location, location) or evening hours or a particular reputed skill or because the guy next door recommends his doctor. And most of the time, if we go to a specialist, we are referred to him or her by another physician whom we trust; we don't cross-examine the referring physician about the specialist's credentials or malpractice experience.

But does this pose an ethics problem? It can, but not because of a lack of free choice. The issue is really how the managed care organization chooses its physicians. Is it strictly on economic performance? Is any physician who is willing to give enough of a discount acceptable? Does the process favor doctors who are so stingy with care that they save huge amounts of money for the HMO, albeit at unacceptable risk to patients? Is the process one of "economic credentialing" (a dreadful term for a dreadful practice), in which profit potential is used as a criterion? Or are stern quality measures, designed to protect patients, used?

A complicating factor is that, at this juncture, most physicians who work in staff- or group-model HMOs—that is, who are on salary or exclusive contracts—are self-selected. They like managed care, they believe in it, and they are good at it. In most cases, they chose it over other forms of practice. Even if they weren't sure about it when they went in, if they are still in it, they have accepted it. Therefore, there is probably a relatively low percentage of HMO physicians who can't tell the difference between conservative care and insufficient care, or who simply can't get with the program.

However, as managed care becomes the dominant mode of healthcare organization—as it likely will—more physicians will be forced into managed care practice who may not understand or accept its principles, the special professional and ethical demands it makes, or the need for vigilance that it entails. Even now, the demand for primary care physicians in the face of a horrendous shortage of those practitioners could tempt HMOs to accept doctors who might be a little marginal. That makes it all the more necessary that the managed care organization be rigorous and unrelenting in developing and enforcing the quality standards it uses in selecting its physician partners.

The other issue here is not original choice of physician but retaining a physician with whom one already has a relationship. We have seen a great deal of disruption as employers and Medicaid programs switch plans and providers, thus breaking up many long-standing physician-patient relationships or else forcing patients to go "out of plan" in order to retain a particular doctor. There's not much to be done about that, and, frankly, we're likely to see a lot more of it.

However, once a patient is in a managed care organization, he or she has every right, in my opinion, to an ongoing relationship with his or her designated primary care physician, obstetrician, and psychiatrist or psychologist. And one should have the same physician throughout a course of treatment for a particular illness or injury. Ethical, high-quality managed care should mean that there is no unnecessary disruption of the patient-physician relationship. That doesn't mean it won't happen; obstetricians can't deliver two babies at once, so if your doctor is busy when you go into labor, you may get another one.

But as a rule, seeking medical care should not be a game of roulette. Constantly switching physicians or making them available on a potluck basis is a violation of one of the basic precepts of managed care, which is the coordination of all services by a single primary care-oriented provider.

Does managed care really involve health maintenance? They are called health maintenance organizations for a reason: They are supposed to be dedicated to early intervention, preventive services, and primary care. Many of them do emphasize these values far more than does the healthcare system as a whole.

On the other hand, many of them do not. In their zest to leverage access, they make early intervention and prevention impossible. One of the most common sins is making patients wait weeks for appointments for a Pap smear, immunization, or cancer screening. Even more awful is making a patient wait weeks for a consultation after a possible malignancy or other serious condition has been detected. That is not managed care; that is abject cruelty.

To the extent that a managed care organization emphasizes (and provides, as opposed to just advertising) timely access to preventive and primary care services, it is operating ethically. To the degree that it makes healthcare an endless waiting game, it is ethically suspect.

I should add that ethical managed care includes proper tending of the mind and spirit. Services such as health promotion instruction, counseling of soon-to-be-discharged patients and the chronically ill, chaplaincy, and, yes, ethics counseling simply must be part of the package.

Indeed, I am particularly worried about the lack of discussion of chaplaincy and spiritual services in the process of promoting managed care and defining "basic benefits." Although I do not belong to an organized religion, I agree with the old saying that there are no atheists in foxholes—and there are few in ICUs. Managed care has an obligation to protect people's hearts and souls as well as their bodies.

Does managed care have social obligations? One bad rap (largely justified) against managed care is that its support of research, health professions education, indigent care, and improvement of community health is notable by its absence. Not only is that often true, but it can be argued that one reason managed care appears to save money (and we don't know for sure that it does) is that it avoids these pursuits and then criticizes the costs of hospitals who do undertake them.

The ethical imperative here is simple: Either the healthcare playing field is going to be level or it isn't. If we are going to excuse managed care from engaging in research, education, social health services, and care of difficult populations, then we must excuse some part of the higher costs of providers who do get involved in these activities.

To me, the more sensible approach is to involve managed care organizations (by force if necessary) in research, education, and universal access. For if they really represent, as they (and I) believe, a superior form of healthcare organization, they should be involved in the training of future physicians and nurses and other professionals, the furthering of the science of healthcare, the improvement of overall health status, and the care of the uninsured poor. Otherwise they are just low-balling their way through society, evading responsibility and making bogus claims of cost-effectiveness.

To their credit, many managed care organizations are aware of these challenges and are trying to address them. There are other guys out there, however, whom we will have to keep an eye on.

The Toad at the Edge of the World

September 1993

See the headnote for "Of Providers and Plagues" (page 14). I would add that this was one of the most controversial columns I ever wrote, and one of those of which I am the most proud.

In *The Green Ripper* by John D. MacDonald, a character likens an impending worldwide disaster to a huge toad perched on the edge of the world, waiting to strike and envelop us all in its horrible maw. . . .

A friend of mine was writing a report on an AIDS conference and was troubled by the lack of interest shown in it by the press. "It's like it's last year's disease," she complained.

She had a point. With the exception of occasional focused coverage of an international AIDS conference, a major report from the Centers for Disease Control, or yet another revelation about the infection or death of a celebrity, we have largely moved on to other things. AIDS and the human immunodeficiency virus (HIV) have become part of the furniture. We are like the people whose hardened faces we see in broadcasts from war zones, talking in flat, matter-of-fact voices about once-unimaginable horrors that are now commonplace.

The Numbers

This journal published a special issue on AIDS in 1987. At the time, there were 15,000 Americans dead of the disease—a shocking figure, I thought. More than 200,000 have died—37,000 this year alone—as of this writing.

There are more than 289,000 known cases in this country and more than 1 million others infected. Worldwide, 14 million people carry the virus: at least 1 million in North America, 1.5 million in Latin America, half a million in western Europe, 75,000 in North Africa and the Middle East (probably under-reported), 8 million in sub-Saharan Africa, 25,000 in Australia and its neighbors, 50,000 in Eastern Europe and Central Asia (probably under-reported), 25,000 in East Asia and the Pacific, and 1.5 million in Southern and Southeast Asia.

In some cities in Asia, 100 percent of the prostitutes are believed to be HIV-positive. In India in 1986, according to a recent *Time* magazine report, there were six reported cases; today, there are a million, expected to rise to 10 million within the decade. As the dreadful trade in forced prostitution and "sex tours" spreads in many parts of the world, the rates will go higher. Some nations in sub-Saharan Africa, an AIDS official told me, are losing their entire professional class.

In eastern Europe, 75 percent of the newly unemployed are women; the *Time* report indicated that a significant number are entering prostitution in their own or neighboring nations. In countries now free but often impoverished, there are few funds for care, let alone prevention. The inevitable is around the corner: Many of those now infected will die without ever having been treated.

Fully 20 million human beings will be infected with this virus by the turn of the century. This is not the type of millennium most of us had in mind.

Tragic Secrecy

Two questions clang like gongs in the face of this: Why do we, in a nation with a much higher per capita rate of infection than many others, still seem unable or unwilling to come to grips with the threat we face? And why, when we do act, are we so stupid about what we do?

It is not like we're short on information, or even on personal experience with the tragedy. A 1993 poll found that 31 percent of Americans know someone who is either sick with or has died of AIDS. In 1987, when we published the special issue of the *Journal*, few people I knew could claim that.

I recall a conversation with a friend who worked in public health; she said she knew no one who had AIDS. I corrected her: "You don't know anyone who has *told you* that he or she has AIDS; I guarantee you know someone who is infected or sick."

How true that was! I spent parts of 1987 and 1988 in New England on an ethics fellowship. When I was getting ready to go home in June 1988, I called my friend Robert (not his real name), who worked in a service business I used, to tell him I was returning and would need his help when I got back. His co-workers told me he was dead. A young man in his thirties, whom I had just seen at Christmas.

What happened? Because his work—which he loved—entailed dealing with the public, he was afraid to tell anyone he was sick, lest he lose his job (and his health insurance). He just extended his Christmas leave and went off and died, alone.

The year that Robert died, Arthur Ashe—Wimbledon champion, international civil rights activist, author, historian, television commentator, former captain of the Davis Cup tennis team—learned he was infected with HIV, the result of a transfusion he had received in 1983 during heart surgery. His last book, completed days before he died of AIDS-related pneumonia on February 6 of this year, is a record of his odyssey as a person with AIDS (*Days of Grace*, Alfred A. Knopf, 1993).

He writes with eloquence about the beginning of that journey: "I cannot say that even the news that I have AIDS devastated me, or drove me into bitter reflection and depression even for a short time. . . . I have been able to stay calm in part because my heart condition is a sufficient source of danger, were I to be terrified by illness.

"My first heart attack, in 1979, could have ended my life in a few chest-ravaging seconds. Both of my heart operations were major surgeries, with the risks attendant on all major surgery. And surely no brain operation is routine [he had brain surgery in 1988 in connection with AIDS-related toxoplasmosis]. Mainly because I have been through these battles with death, I have lost much of my fear of it."

Yet he feared something else. This American hero—a champion revered both by the world of sports and the larger society—kept his condition secret. This was due in part, he tells us, to an utterly justified desire for privacy, but another part of it was a terror that he would be ruined, professionally and financially, if people learned about his condition.

He was able to keep his secret until someone—he did not know who—tipped off the press. A close friend of his, a reporter, was assigned the dreadful task of finding out if it was true. Although he refused to answer the question, Ashe knew the story would be released, and so, on April 8, 1992, he revealed the news at a press conference.

Even then, as an internationally renowned author and activist, he feared being dropped from his board memberships and having endorsement and consulting contracts cancelled and speaking invitations withdrawn. He was enormously grateful when these things did not happen.

My God, what have we come to in this country?

Item: Bill Clinton, the president who ran on a platform of change and conciliation, promised to allow Haitians fleeing the brutality of a military dictatorship refuge in this country. Instead, he continued his predecessor's policy of turning them back—and then allowed those found to have legitimate claims of persecution, but who were HIV-positive, to remain incarcerated in a glorified concentration camp at Guantanamo Bay, where they had been for nearly two years, until a federal judge freed them.

(In 14th-century Genoa, a boatload of Genoese infected with Black Plague was turned away from the harbor by the city fathers; as a result, it had to land at another port, from which the disease spread rapidly into central Europe. Genoa itself, despite its precautions, suffered a full measure of plague.)

This past June, Clinton signed a bill continuing the U.S. ban on entry into the country by HIV-infected persons.

Item: The U.S. Supreme Court, on November 9, 1992, in what has become known as the McGann decision, upheld the right of a self-insured employer to retroactively deny health benefits to an employee with AIDS. Jack McGann, a music company worker in Houston, Texas, found that he had the disease; his employer, H & H Music Company, told him that instead of the $1 million in benefits he was told he would have as an employee when he joined the firm, his benefits were capped at $5,000.

(The Equal Employment Opportunity Commission has now ruled, in the case of a construction worker with AIDS who, like Jack McGann, found his benefits retroactively terminated, that persons with AIDS are disabled and are therefore protected by the Americans with Disabilities Act. They thus usually cannot be denied coverage. It will be interesting to see if this decision is widely enforced.)

Item: As of this writing, 70 percent of AIDS patients in this country do not have private insurance; most of those who have any coverage at all are on Medicaid. In 1989, of the 25,126 AIDS patients who were cared for by a surveyed group of 526 hospitals, 71 percent were treated in public hospitals, which represented only 20 percent of the hospitals in the survey.

A 1991 survey found that among gay male and leukemia patients in Baltimore and Los Angeles, 90 percent of those without AIDS had private coverage, whereas only 64 percent of persons with AIDS did. Individuals with AIDS were 33 times as likely as those with other illnesses to be on Medicaid, and five times as likely to have lost private insurance.

(In a recent, despondent article on the swath that AIDS has cut through the arts community, *Newsweek* noted that there's a reason so many recent Broadway musical hits have been revivals: Most of a generation of choreographers, who would have created new works, are dead.

On the cover of that issue was a glorious portrait of Rudolf Nureyev, also dead of AIDS. He asked that the cause of his death be concealed; he didn't want people to know.)

Enough Is Enough

At some point, you stop and say, enough is enough. For me, it was Arthur Ashe's death. His is a tale of good intentions gone wrong. He admits, in his book, that the transfusion that ended up killing him was optional, and that it was his choice to have it. But he was long since reconciled to that maddening fact: "I was simply unlucky enough to have had a couple of units of transfused blood that may have been donated in 1983 by some gay or bisexual man, or some intravenous drug user who perhaps had needed the money badly. I will never know for sure, and this is not an issue I dwell on."

He goes on to say that he was blessed with money, familial support, three health insurance policies, excellent healthcare, previous experience with serious illness, and a capacity for coping. He mourns the fact that most of those with AIDS do not have that kind of protection.

What nearly undid him was the rape-like violation of his privacy by a news organization that had been tipped off, in all likelihood, by a healthcare worker. He points out that it is widely known that healthcare workers are paid by "news" organizations to be on the lookout for such tidbits. He asks for a higher level of decency than that from us.

Now he is gone, along with millions of others around the world.

Two Little Girls

Our failure to come to grips with AIDS can be told in the differing stories of two little girls. One is six-year-old Camera Ashe, the daughter of Jeanne Moutoussamy and Arthur Ashe. She is, fortunately, free of HIV infection, as is her mother.

Her late father said, in a speech at the United Nations on World AIDS Day in 1992: "We must try and we must succeed, or our children and grandchildren will one day rightfully ask us why, in the face of such a calamity, we did not give our best efforts. What shall we tell them—and their mothers in particular—if we don't measure up? How shall I answer my six-year-old daughter, and what do we say to the estimated 10 million AIDS orphans by the year 2000?"

There was another little girl, who will not be among those orphans, although she might have been. Her name was Jackie Johnson, and she, too, was six years old. She lived in Florida, and she killed herself in June of this year by standing in front of a train. Her brother and cousins tried to pull her away, but she refused their help. The news reports said she was despondent because her mother was dying of AIDS.

Her name will not appear in the *Morbidity and Mortality Weekly Report;* there will be no square for her in the AIDS quilt. But AIDS killed her, all the same.

We owed Jackie hope, and we failed her; we owe Camera a future, and we can still give her that.

But it will be no picnic. Humankind is facing a holocaust as grim as those perpetrated by the Nazis, by Pol Pot and the Khmer Rouge, and by the ethnic cleansers of Bosnia. It does not matter whether its victims are Zambians or New Yorkers, gays or infants, the wealthy or the weak; it's too late for the making of fine and meaningless distinctions.

The AIDS community knows this. One of the loudest voices of protest over the internment of HIV-positive Haitians at Guantanamo was that of the Gay Men's Health Crisis organization in New York City. Shortly before he died, Arthur Ashe was arrested while picketing the White House in support of the Haitians.

The global village is not the newly minted product of faster electronic communications or more airplanes or CNN. It has always been here; we have always shared this earth, all of one species, all brothers and sisters. We have no other place to call home, no other biological family to which we belong. E.E. Cummings wrote it: "I am also a you."

That toad at the edge of the world is there now, waiting. It is a retrovirus that is spread through sexual contact, infected blood, exchange of certain bodily fluids, ignorance, fear, and hatred. It could swallow the new freedom of eastern Europe, the blossoming economies of the Pacific Rim, the ancient societies of Africa, and the United States of America.

We must look it in the face and say, "You will go no further." We must embrace each other in the face of this monster and the monsters it breeds within us, and say, "It stops here." We must do this, all of us, on behalf of all of us, or else the monster will win.

· · · · · · ·

Some Frank Advice

The AIDS pandemic has killed four times as many Americans as died in Vietnam. I have, therefore, decided that it is time to stop being polite. Arthur Ashe wrote of the kind of sex education that is necessary: It may not be the typical discussion topic in polite society, "but there is nothing polite about AIDS."

So let me be impolite. Here is some frank advice.

To healthcare providers:

- *If you don't want to treat patients with this illness, get out of healthcare. Many provider organizations have made this a matter of policy, and they are right. Healthcare is an odd line of work for those who don't want to be around sick people.*

- *Take seriously the precautions that can save your life and those of others; learn the nature of the disease and its transmission, and stop taking short cuts because you find protecting yourself or others time-consuming or inconvenient. Insist that your*

employers provide the time and resources for inservice education about this virus and the diseases it causes.

If you see other providers engaging in unsafe practices that
endanger them or patients, call them on it. With the exception
of dentist David Acer in Florida and whatever he was up to,
we do not have firm evidence of provider-to-patient transmission of HIV. Let's try to keep it that way.

- If your employers or insurers make even the slightest move toward
denying or reducing benefits to co-workers who develop AIDS,
go public with the information (without violating the AIDS
patient's privacy) and shame them into rescinding the decision.

- Treat information about the HIV status of a patient as though it
were information about you or a loved one. The confidentiality
of any such information is sacred. If, in this age of data and computerization, you think your organization has not implemented
sufficient safeguards for patient information, complain about it.

    Insist that the critical importance of the confidentiality of
patient information be part of all training and continuing education throughout the organization. If you know of a healthcare worker who is feeding information to the press or to
insurers, turn him or her in.

- Support your co-workers and colleagues who are working with
HIV-infected patients. I hear stories of burnout; of broken
hearts because a favorite patient died; of frustration and rage
because an HIV-infected woman has gotten pregnant—again;
of horror at men with AIDS who knowingly, even intentionally, impregnate women and then abandon them. Those who
care for these very sick people are quiet heroes and heroines
among us, and they deserve our admiration and support.

To trustees and other community leaders:

- Offer both treatment and prevention, and do not support policies that lead to avoiding patients simply because they have HIV

disease. Support community education programs, including frank discussions of sexual practices and drug use. Bring in a speaker who has AIDS to talk to community organizations, your employees, your church congregation, your children's classes.

- Support prevention among addicts, including the use of bleach and condoms—and needle exchange programs. This is a tough issue for me. As a former drug counselor who knows first-hand the disaster that drug use often produces, I have been uneasy with needle exchange, viewing it as a virtual abandonment of the drug-using population in favor of just trying to contain the disease, a form of "don't get your cooties on me."

  But we are past such niceties of philosophy now. I was instructed in this by Pam Lichty, then head of the governor's AIDS commission in Hawaii, who pointed out that a goodly number of addicts who participate in needle exchange programs end up seeking treatment, which is the ultimate goal.

- While you're at it, support effective addiction treatment, by which I mean proven programs that are culturally appropriate to the population, not boutique for-profit yuppie drug treatment programs that are most notable for their high costs and higher rates of recidivism.

To politicians and policymakers:

- Support treatment and prevention programs with the same enthusiasm with which you are pouring millions of dollars into sometimes questionable research efforts.

- Demand more accountability of researchers; the growing scandal surrounding the National Institutes of Health scientists who claim to have discovered the AIDS virus and the blood test for it is a grotesque reminder that this area of research, like others, has its cesspools of profiteering and unconscionable selfishness.

  Keep in mind the French health officials who knowingly allowed tainted blood to be distributed because they wanted the French to develop their own blood test (and besides, it would be such a waste to throw out all that blood). They have since been convicted of criminal behavior; 15,000 French people now are infected with HIV courtesy of that little exercise in national pride and cost-effectiveness.

- Face the bigots, the reactionaries, the holier-than-thou demagogues with their smug beliefs about queers and junkies and hookers—and spit in their eye. No epidemic in history has ever confined itself to the group in which it began; no virus has yet conducted a means test or exercised a moral judgment before it attacked. Viruses don't come with religious beliefs.

  The job of the public official is to protect the public health, and the public health is the health of all of us, no matter who we are. Do your job; if more public officials had been willing to do so while Ronald Reagan and his friends were pretending nothing was wrong, we would not be in the desperate straits we are in today.

- Support and implement insurance underwriting reforms that prevent commercial and nonprofit carriers alike from disenfranchising the HIV population and those at risk of joining it.

  Support universal access to coverage and care for all, including those tens of millions of people too poor to acquire their own policies. State Medicaid programs are cracking under the strain; Medicaid spending went up 25 percent last year, partially because it has become the primary insurance program for persons with AIDS.

  Force the insurers to do what the public expects them to do: Cover the sick. If they are unwilling to provide coverage to those with HIV, tell them they can no longer sell insurance in your state. Support the Congressional action that will be needed to prevent self-insured employers from jettisoning HIV-infected workers.

To each of you as parents, citizens, and Americans:

- Wear a red ribbon. It provides many opportunities for discussing the epidemic and what needs to be done. Donate time or money to an AIDS cause. Cook dinner for a sick friend and take it over to him or her. Go cuddle an orphaned baby with AIDS, as the members of the League of 100 Black Women in Washington, DC do.

- Put a package of condoms and the frankest AIDS education materials you can find in your kid's top drawer or purse or wallet, and in the suitcase when he or she goes away to school or on holiday. Do the same for your spouse or lover. (I once gave condoms to a man I loved for his birthday. I hoped he would never be in a situation when he needed to use them, but I would rather he did than risk himself or me.)

A dear friend of mine, a veteran of the Sixties, as I am, recently sat down with her beautiful teenaged children, and said: "I am sorry, in some ways, that you cannot engage in the sexual experimentation I did when I was young. It is tantalizing and thrilling for people of your age. But you can't; it could kill you."

Like her, I would like to think that my young friends know that abstinence and development of a long-term, mutually monogamous relationship with a single individual are the best ways to protect oneself. But unlike her, I am not willing to believe that all the young ones I know will follow that route.

Thus, when friends young or old or in-between talk of a new relationship, I ask: Has he/she been tested for HIV? Have you? Are you using condoms? Are you using them correctly and effectively? Is there anything you want to know about AIDS? What do you know about it?

And I have told many of my friends who have young children that I would like them to give the kids my name and phone number; if they need to talk to someone who is not a parent and who will respect their privacy, I want to be available.

• • • • • • •

My honorarium for this column was donated to the Arthur Ashe Endowment for the Defeat of AIDS, c/o Dr. Henry Murray, Box 130, New York Hospital, 525 E. 68th Street, New York, NY 10021.

An Ounce of Compassion

November 1993

A great many things changed in this country during the Seventies and Eighties, from our level of debt as a nation to how we treat our bodies. Indeed, according to Humphrey Taylor, president of Louis Harris Associates, more of us began exercising regularly, quitting cigarettes, and eating less fat- and cholesterol-laden foods. "Mainly as a result of these lifestyle changes," Taylor writes in *Health Management Quarterly* (Second Quarter 1992), "the incidence of heart disease (while still the nation's No. 1 killer) has fallen dramatically and life expectancy has steadily improved."

He goes on, "Americans are the world's supreme optimists, and most of us assume that those improvements will go on, if not forever, at least for the next few decades and that we will all become more faithful disciples of Jane Brody, exercising more and eating more wisely."

If this were to be the case, it would mark an extraordinary change in how Americans view health and healthcare; it would mean that we have exchanged one god for another.

In his landmark book, *The Mirage of Health* (Anchor Books, 1959), Nobel laureate Rene Dubos described the Greek myths of Hygeia and Asclepius as symbols of "the never-ending oscillation between two different points of view in medicine. For the worshipers of Hygeia [the goddess thought to protect the health of Athenians], health is the natural order of things, a positive attribute to which men are entitled if they govern their lives wisely. According to them, the most important function of medicine is to discover and teach the natural laws which will ensure to man a healthy mind in a healthy body."

On the other hand, followers of Asclepius, who legend says was Greece's first physician, "believe that the chief role of the physician is to treat disease, to restore health by correcting any imperfection caused by the accidents of birth or life," according to Dubos.

In the battle between these two ideals, Dubos concludes that "to ward off disease or recover health, men as a rule find it easier to depend on healers than to attempt the more difficult task of living wisely."

It thus should not be surprising that, despite Simplesse and Soloflex, nicotine patches and Nautilus, Taylor reports that the Harris Prevention Index, which has tracked the spread of healthy habits since 1983, shows that things improved until 1987, but little has been gained since.

Although we are using auto seat belts and smoke detectors more, and are driving while intoxicated somewhat less, the decline in smoking has been only one-half of 1 percent per year since 1983; the big gain was between 1975 and 1983. And Taylor observes that "all the hype about fitness and nutrition has more to do with aspirations and with marketing than with reality."

"Public Health Fascism"

Yet despite this evidence, the philosophy spreading like a brush fire is that if we just do enough push-ups, eat enough fish, abjure all our enjoyable but harmful habits, and drive responsibly, we will save huge amounts of money, will never have to "ration" health services, and will all look like Cindy Crawford (or Marky Mark, or whoever your ideal of fitness is).

Accompanying this classically naive expression of American optimism is a disdain for those who don't get with the program.

"Couch potatoes" are a lower form of life. People with alcohol or other drug dependencies are weak. Overweight individuals (especially women) are denigrated, desexualized, and discriminated against. Nicotine addicts are learning to live under rocks—and the rocks are probably complaining loudly about second-hand smoke. Our growing obsession with prevention has given rise to an attitude that professor George Annas of Boston University describes as "public health fascism."

Meanwhile, there is a great deal of money to be made, from Jenny Craig to World Gym to the substance abuse treatment industry. The number of products that are missing something—salt, sugar, fat, cholesterol, preservatives, what have you—is growing exponentially. (I always worry about what they replace those things with, but we'll go into that another time.)

It seems that the prevention movement is in danger of losing its way. If it does, it won't be the first time.

Before the Fifties, public and preventive health measures saved millions of lives through cleaner food and water, purer air, immunization, safer childbirth, and community nursing. Indeed, public health nursing was once the most prestigious branch of the profession, and its practitioners enjoyed the greatest degree of autonomy of any nurses in history. Sadly, it lost its position on that pinnacle, as did public health generally.

Today, Hygeia and Asclepius continue to battle for the hearts and minds of the American people, but their relationship is getting stranger by the minute. On the one hand, the popular culture, advertising, and societal norms have embraced the image of the lean, yogurt-swilling, nonsmoking, American long-distance runner as the ideal.

On the other hand, as of this writing, most health insurance does not sufficiently cover preventive services, if they are covered at all. Pregnancy often requires a rider on a policy, and Medicare only got around to covering mammography in the past two years. "The big money is in diagnosis and treatment, not prevention," writes Taylor. "So providers and the healthcare industry have little real interest in fighting for money for prevention."

Indeed, the heart of the acute-care sector lies with Asclepius. Providers can take more than a little share of the blame for the relegation of preventive health services to second-class citizenship in the land of healthcare.

Prevention is at a crossroads. It is being promoted as the answer to skyrocketing healthcare costs, and touted as the linchpin of managed care. On the other hand, we are not pursuing it as vigorously as the advertising barons would have us believe, perhaps because it's hard to find the time, money, and commitment. And we certainly are not paying for it in terms of third-party coverage or funding for public health.

So perhaps we should ask: What is it we are trying to prevent? The prevention of needless disease, disability, and death has become tangled up with other, less laudable beliefs in our society, and, as a fervent exponent of preventive care, I would like to try to tease some of those tangles out.

What Is the Goal of Prevention?

Preventive and public health services were once community-oriented, as opposed to person-oriented. That is, if the water had cyanide in it, the entire community was threatened. Polio could hit anybody. The ban-the-bomb movement of the Fifties was a form of preventive health activity, because the use of nuclear or biological weapons threatens the entire earth. (Nevil Shute's *On the Beach*, a chronicle of the last survivors of a meaningless atomic war that destroyed the world, remains one of the most horrifying books one could ever read.)

But community-oriented preventive health may have been killed by its own success. As I have observed before, the best public health department is marked by the absence of ill health or environmental disaster. The most successful preventive services are those whose evidence is the absence of disease. The savings are hard to document, and too often the funding gets cut.

So while community-oriented prevention has taken hit after hit, we have seen the rise of person-oriented prevention. It is a different critter. It is generally not a public service, but rather a private one, and highly profitable at that. And its gospel is that the only thing that matters is individual effort.

The remnants of community orientation are seen in the well-worn (and absolutely true) argument that prevention saves society money. Of course it does. The measles that don't occur, the cancer that is not contracted, the *salmonella* that doesn't show up in the fast food are all expenses that were not incurred.

But we don't know how to do the accounting—and the price has to be paid months, years, or decades before the payoff. (For example, how many public health departments, by refusing to issue permits, prevented the kind of toxic pollution that destroyed the Love Canal community in New York? Did they get any points for that?)

But the argument that prevention's main (or only) virtue is that it saves money seems misguided. This was eloquently argued by Henry Aaron, of the Brookings Institution, at the June 1993 meeting of the Association for Health Services Research. Listening to yet another plea for funding of preventive care because it saves money, Aaron replied that he was uncomfortable with prevention for children being portrayed solely as a big cost-saver. To paraphrase his outburst: "The reason for providing these services is that we want healthy, happy children, not simply that it saves money. We should want to achieve that whether it saves money or not."

We should pursue prevention, not simply because it saves society money (which is true), or that it costs less than other kinds of health services (which is true), or that it produces a healthier workforce (which is true). We should engage in preventive services because they give people a better life, which is part and parcel of the American dream.

And that means giving community-oriented prevention as much of a place at the table as the person-oriented, glitzy preventions of the Nineties, which fewer and fewer of us can afford, and whose iffy outcomes lead me to wonder whether we are preventing ill health, or promoting high incomes for those who are expert in exploiting what Taylor refers to as "aspirations and marketing."

Death Is Not Optional

I think of four friends. Two are thin, physically active vegetarians, one of whom has a cholesterol count around 300. The other just had bypass surgery. A third had a coronary while jogging. The fourth leads an almost monkish life—no alcohol, meat, or drugs— and is in perfect health other than the fact that he is HIV-positive.

Dubos reminds us, "Life is like a large body of water moved by deep currents and by superficial breezes. We have gained some understanding of the winds and can adjust our sails to them. But the really powerful forces that determine population trends are deep currents of which we know little, the fundamental physical and biological laws of the world, the habits and beliefs of mankind with their roots deep in the past."

We still don't know why most smokers don't get lung cancer, why athletes die on the field while nonathletes live to 103. We have our beliefs and our judgments, and we run from oat bran to niacin to biofeedback, trying to gain control of the unknown.

But the fact is, Dubos cautions, that "the use of knowledge must be tempered by humility and commonsense, and for this reason medical utopias must be taken with a great deal of salt." (Oh, all right—we'll take them with a great deal of salt substitute.) He believed that humankind's efforts to combat nature, environment, and fate "will often result in failure, partial or total, temporary or permanent. Disease will remain an inescapable manifestation of [people's] struggles."

In other words, we're all going to die of something.

George Annas has said that contemporary medicine sometimes seems to evince the belief that "death is an optional event." It is not.

The best—the very best—that prevention can buy us is a longer time of good health. That is not a shabby goal; indeed, most of us would take a few years less on this earth in good, functional health in exchange for a few more years of dysfunction. But in the end, we will have to take what we are dealt, and can only work to make the most of those cards.

What If You Can't?

I have been troubled for years by a deodorant commercial (I am troubled by all deodorant commercials, but we'll go into that another time as well) that says, "All you have to do is give 110 percent."

Great. What if you have cystic fibrosis? What if you are missing a limb? What if you are plagued by profound depression?

What if your self-esteem has been shattered? This, to me, is the single most powerful obstacle faced by the prevention movement. Your husband just left you for a younger, slimmer woman. Your child has AIDS. You just lost your job. You are stopped by the police nightly because you happen to be young, male, and African-American.

How much guts does it take to go to the gym (if you can afford it), to find the time to run, to not turn to nicotine or alcohol or Valium or cocaine? People who are fragile enough, or get hit often enough, or are alone and unsupported enough, give up. On wellness. On prevention. And on themselves.

There are a whole lot of reasons why people can't live up to what we expect of them. Sure, some of the problem is laziness, self-indulgence, or ignorance. But a lot more of it is genes, the enormous differences among people in terms of how much good preventive activity does, and cultural differences in a society in which white, upper-middle-class norms are laid on people who live in very different ways. Indeed, the health promotion movement sometimes smacks of the kind of intolerant messianic zeal that led the Spaniards to dispatch the Incas and their magnificent civilization simply because it was different and they didn't understand it.

Do I pursue health promotion myself? You bet. I aspire to exercise every day, and on most days I make it. I don't use illegal drugs or nicotine or coffee. (I do drink tea and wine.) Raised on a cuisine that was half-Jewish and half-Southern, I now duly subscribe to the gospel of chicken breasts, salad, and other sometimes-boring things, and it is only rarely that I give in to my fantasies about fried chicken wings, corned beef sandwiches, and biscuits with gravy.

But I also know that my fate may have been largely determined before I was born, and that the stress of my work may undo much of the halibut and the miles and the laps. I weigh too much, I am stressed out, and I use caffeine and alcohol. And I fear being stomped on by a society that is notoriously intolerant, and that may have found, in prevention, an entirely new way to be intolerant. As Roger Evans, a humane and astute observer, has written of the uninsured poor, "Their plight reflects the unwillingness of our sociopolitical system to reward failure" (*Health Management Quarterly,* Second Quarter 1992).

If prevention is the new god, there is a new devil as well: the person who gets fat, or flabby, or addicted, or sick anyway. Evans warns us: "As we pursue the ideology of preventive health, those persons who have inherited or acquired health deficiencies (for which they are considered responsible) will necessarily be viewed as pariahs who place excessive demands on society."

There, with or without the grace of God, may go I.

What Happens If We Succeed?

Among the consequences of success in prevention could be the fiscal failure of many healthcare reform schemes that are financed through "sin taxes" on alcohol, tobacco, and (one hopes) firearms. (I heartily support such taxes, by the way.) If we all stop smoking, drinking, and shooting, the healthcare system could collapse for lack of funds (and acute patients)!

But I wouldn't count on it. Even if we do stop smoking, drinking, and shooting, we will still need a healthcare system. We can prevent all kinds of things, but there are many things we cannot prevent. And the ones we can't prevent are tougher than they used to be. To quote William Campbell, MD, a St. Louis physician, "Let's face it; most of the cheap and easy diseases have been taken care of."

If we prevent acute childhood illness and injury, and adolescent conditions (especially sexually transmitted diseases, AIDS, and gunshot wounds), and unnecessary adult health problems, we will all get old, and a goodly percentage of us will become chronically ill. Some of us will be chronically ill much earlier than that.

I have to wonder what will become of us old farts with unexotic diabetes and glaucoma and COPD and general wearing-out. We fear being unable to see or hear or smell or walk well, because this society has little use for the profoundly disabled or "feeble." We fear being removed from society into nursing homes that resemble senior ghettos (although not all of them are).

I fear becoming such an exile; I bet you do, too.

Ethicist Daniel Callahan says he thinks that much of the fear of dying in this country has to do with a fear of abandonment—of being left to die alone. Because of this terror, we demand that the healthcare system stay with us, and we carry this demand even to the point of useless existence-prolonging technology. Callahan has therefore suggested that the highest healthcare priority should be caring and comfort for those who cannot get well.

Yet our current healthcare system often abandons the chronically ill and dying. They do not represent success. Jenny Craig cannot narrate their stories on television; they cannot endorse running shoes. No one can use them to make the rest of us feel inadequate because they have achieved perfect health and we have not.

And so we abandon them—and then wonder in disbelief as they demand "the works" and insist that they are not dying, that there is still hope, that they can be cured. If there is any time in life when one needs one's personhood reinforced, it is when he or she is disabled or dying. But if the gods of prevention view the sick as failures, and the healthcare system resents their presence, what are they to do?

A Safe Haven

Prevention, in the end, is a limited means to a limited end. Within those limits—genes, personal ability, culture, money, chance, and commitment—it can make for a better life. But it will not keep us from getting sick, and, in the end, dying.

In old Hawaii, there was a place called the Puuhonua O Honaunau—the Place of Refuge. Back when the Hawaiians warred frequently against each other, and when *kapus* (taboos) were common, this was safe haven. Even if you had fought for the wrong side, or had broken a *kapu*, or had otherwise offended the gods, if you could somehow make it inside the walls of the Puuhonua O Honaunau, you were safe. A *kahuna* (priest) would dress your wounds, absolve you of your sins, and send you on your way, forgiven.

I was recently told by an acquaintance about King Leopold's Fountain, in Vienna. He said that in the old days, those convicted of crimes would be allowed to go free if they could make it to the fountain and touch it. I told him about the Place of Refuge, and we decided that every culture must have a deep need to see itself as at least a little forgiving. Every culture has a small corner that offers sanctuary.

Healthcare must be a place of sanctuary. Even as we strive to help people live healthier lives, we must be a place where those who have lost the race for health can come in safety, a place without judgmentalism, condemnation, or hatred.

Yes, we must prevent those conditions we can prevent. Yes, we should treat our minds and bodies better. But we must also forgive, and continue to provide safe haven for those who are sick and broken. Pain, fear, illness, injury, and death are punishment enough.

Don't Do Her Wrong

January 1994

Women's healthcare—that is, services specifically directed to female patients—has become a booming business in recent years. Dedicated women's programs, women's centers, disease-specific efforts focusing on breast cancer and endometriosis, and many other initiatives have proven both popular and profitable.

It was a market waiting to be found. Of the 76 million baby boomers, more than half are women, and 90 percent had been born when Betty Friedan published *The Feminine Mystique*. A great many were influenced by the women's movement and by feminist healthcare organizations such as the Boston Women's Health Book Collective.

As these autonomy-seeking women encountered traditional medicine—which was often male-dominated, institution-dominated, technology-dominated, and paternalistic—the resultant clash of values opened up a marketing niche the size of the Grand Canyon, and made women's healthcare an easy sell (to patients, if not to the provider establishment). In record time, we went from informal rap groups in college dorms to women's centers where every inch is designed to attract disaffected women patients.

That these centers have provided a more accessible and user-friendly environment for women patients is obvious. But there is in the women's health movement a risk of substituting form for substance. Dusty-rose curtains and turquoise couches, an all-female staff, and an emphasis on privacy and sensitivity appeal to women who are weary of a healthcare system that at times resembles an assembly line. Unfortunately, the attractive trappings can also hide poor quality of care, questionable appropriateness, inefficiency, squandered resources, and violation of patients' rights—not through a hard sell, but through a soft one. Having pink curtains does not mean that we automatically deserve patients' trust.

So there are ethics questions that are specific to women's health-care. Some involve internal issues within a program; others are external and have to do with the relationship of the center or pro-gram to the rest of the world. These issues affect two groups: staff members and patients. Here are some of these questions.

How well are nonprofessional staff members treated? It's a good guess that the vast majority of them are women; does the environment of tolerance, sensitivity, and, most important, equity apply to them?

Is childcare provided? If it is, can anyone except the medical and top administrative staff afford it? Most lower-echelon healthcare workers are women with younger children and are often single mothers to boot; this is also true of many nurses. Do staffing pat-terns and employee benefits accommodate their specific needs?

In too many healthcare settings where the patients are treated like royalty, the nonmedical staff are treated like lower forms of life—especially if they are women.

Is there a mechanism for staff to bring ethics dilemmas to the attention of the leadership? If there is a problem, do staff feel comfortable "blowing the whistle," or do they feel that they may do the right thing at the cost of their jobs?

A survey conducted a few years ago by Judith M. Wilkinson, RN, examined the ethics problems nurses face. (See "Moral Distress in Nursing," by Donald F. Phillips, in *Choices and Conflict: Explorations in Health Care Ethics*, American Hospital Publishing, 1992.) The respondents reported that many of their most awful dilemmas involved witnessing malpractice, excessive care, skimpy care, violation of patients' rights, treatment without patient permission, and the like. Could such things be going on in your setting?

Do women's health professionals advocate for women within the organization? I don't mean soliciting a budget increase to buy mauve curtains to replace the dusty-rose ones. I mean advocating for all staff members. Every year, a few women night-shift workers are murdered while hiking out to parking places that are beyond the Back Forty. Training and advancement opportunities for low-echelon workers are often hard to come by, even with some two dozen healthcare professions in short supply. And, needless to say, the continuing lack of women in CEO and board leadership positions sends messages to female employees about their relative worth—and prospects—within the organization.

And what happens to patients when their care extends beyond the women's center? Is every woman patient who is referred for inpatient care tracked to ensure that the promised environment of support and sensitivity is carried over? Does the women's center push energetically for a continuum of care for patients throughout the organization?

And, perhaps most important in the me-first times in which we live, do women's healthcare professionals share the lessons they've learned with the rest of the organization, so that their successes—and failures—can be used to improve the care of all patients, men and women alike?

Are women being over-treated? In terms of quality, there is an enormous opportunity for women's health professionals to provide poor care. In 1989, a survey by the National Association of Women's Health Professionals found that the greatest challenge cited by members was "building volume for services." Women's centers, like any other program, have to justify their existence and their budgets, especially these days. And in women's care, as elsewhere in healthcare, we may believe we are providing perfectly appropriate care, without realizing we are way over the line.

Example: A report by Martin L. Brown and others in the October 1, 1990, *Annals of Internal Medicine* found that the United States had four times as many mammography machines as would be needed, by any measure, to screen women for breast cancer. The number of machines rose from 134 in 1982 to 8,000 in 1988 and is higher now. The researchers predicted—correctly—that this excess would inevitably produce high prices that would prevent many women from getting the procedure. Even with the advent of Medicare payment for mammography (which, incredibly, only occurred in the past three years), many women at high risk of disease are not being screened. This is a market run amok.

Overcapacity (and its attendant temptations) is only one part of the overselling of health services to women. In scanning newspapers and magazines—especially the women's sections—one can see that advertisements playing on women's health fears are commonplace. As managed care takes hold while overcapacity lingers, we could see ads declaring that women should get two mammograms a year, or three—even in the face of recommendations to the contrary by research organizations.

And why not? Already there are extensive ads in every Sunday newspaper supplement for procedures to remove spider veins, enlarge or reduce breasts, suck fat, and make other helpful contributions to support the culture of inadequacy that continues to terrorize American women.

As providers of women's healthcare, our procedures, our recommendations, and our protocols must be rooted in outcomes research, databased quality assessment, and standards for appropriateness. Caregivers should not play on fear; just because a market for the unnecessary exists does not mean we should pander to it.

This commitment is especially needed in light of the fact that as women age in this unforgiving culture, they can become more and more paranoid about their appearance, their health, and their aging. They can easily be put on a treadmill of constant cosmetic surgery, dubious psychological therapy, and overcare.

Are women denied needed care? But this sword has two edges. As managed care becomes more and more dominant, the other edge begins to show. The temptation at the other end of the spectrum is to deny needed services because of the financial incentives involved in managed care, about which I have written in previous columns. To me, proper managed care means coordination of all services by a primary-care provider; it is based on notions of integration, continuum, and appropriateness. Unfortunately, to many others, managed care is a dandy way to make money denying needed care to people. As was noted in the October 12, 1993 issue of *USA Today* (page 10A), there is nothing to stop an unscrupulous HMO from recruiting patients, signing them up, taking their money (or that of their sponsors)—and then taking its phone off the hook.

Indeed, recently I saw an unacceptable bit of managed care from a for-profit HMO: a preprinted slip of paper, mailed without comment in an envelope, that read, "The results of your Pap smear . . . indicate a need for re-testing in three months. If you have any questions, please call the OB/GYN department." Even to an educated, consumerist patient, that would be terrifying, but for any patient, it represents a form of abandonment.

The ethics of quality of care for women or anybody else are straightforward: Provide what the patient needs. Not more. Not less. And if we don't know what the patient needs, we must actively participate in research that will tell us.

Are women's healthcare programs overly selective? Women's programs usually target the best-insured and most socially acceptable patients. The result is that when less socially attractive patients find their way to us, we may—consciously or not—treat them with something less than the sensitivity promised on the shingle hanging outside the door.

One group at particular risk of discrimination is the chronically ill, whom providers have been shunning for 300 years. It's no wonder; our healthcare system has always been based on acute care of the curable. The chronically ill, the dying, and the mad used to be shunted away to the almshouse; today it is too often the nursing home, the attic, or, in the case of our still brutal treatment of the chronically mentally ill, the sidewalk.

Women's centers have not focused on the demographic reality: The best way to ensure yourself a spot in the healthcare system of the 21st century is to have a program that attracts little old ladies with chronic conditions. Infertility programs may be all the rage, but remember that in another 15 years, most baby boom women will be past childbearing age. Furthermore, few reform proposals include coverage for expensive infertility treatments.

A much better bet is expert care of arthritis. Alzheimer's disease. Incontinence. We should be planning to provide what the women of this country are going to need. And if you are horrified by the prospect of a patient population that is more Grumpie (Art Hoppe's description of aging boomers as Grown-Up Mature People) than Yuppie, you need a little attitude adjustment.

But it is not just a problem for the aging and the chronically ill. Take the case of the addicted mother. She is an easy target. One's blood rises in anger that someone would abuse her unborn child. The image that the press has so enthusiastically hurled at us comes into focus: poor, minority, uncaring, using drugs for kicks.

I remind you of an article I have quoted before in this column— by Ira Chasnoff, MD, and his colleagues (*New England Journal of Medicine*, April 26, 1990), who explored the reporting of pregnant women showing evidence of drug use to authorities in Pinellas County, Florida. The authors took the urine of every pregnant woman seeking prenatal care in private physicians' offices or in public clinics in that part of Florida for one month, and then followed up on how many were found to have been using drugs or alcohol— and how many of these were turned in to the local or state authorities under state law requiring such reporting.

The rate of drug or alcohol use, overall, was between 14 and 15 percent for black and white women alike; there was no statistical difference. Black women used cocaine more often; white women used cannabis drugs more often. But the same proportion of each group tested positive. As a woman physician observed about the findings, it is not a question of race. If you're not finding drug-exposed babies except among the poor and minority groups, you're not looking very hard for them.

But the really troubling finding was that black women found to have used drugs in pregnancy were ten times more likely to be turned in to the authorities as white women. And low-income women were more likely than middle- or upper-income women to be turned in.

There's a great line from an old (1931) movie about newspaper abuse of people's privacy and its tragic results. At one point, a secretary, futilely opposing a newspaper's intention to dig up and republish nasty details about a prominent woman's former life, sighs and concedes, "You can always get people interested in the crucifixion of a woman."

Certainly that is true if she is pregnant and addicted, especially if she is black. And the states respond. In South Carolina, addicted women were arrested and handcuffed to their hospital beds the day they gave birth. Another woman was placed under house arrest for two months before she gave birth.

We are sympathetic to the bulimic and the anorexic and contemptuous of the obese. We cater to the marginally depressed and we flee from the seriously mentally ill. We pity the middle-class cocaine user in her suburban home, but we arrest the crack user.

This is inequity, plain and simple. It is rife in healthcare, as it is rife in society. Women's healthcare should be a refuge from it.

What about women and suicide? Let us leave aside for now the fact that some patients would rather kill themselves than submit to our ministrations and what that implies about how we have organized our oncology and hospice services. The main point is that Jack Kevorkian (rightly described by ethicist Arthur Caplan as a "serial mercy killer") has now participated in the deaths of nearly 20 people—most of them sick, aging women.

It is ironic, scary, and unfortunately historically consistent that little fuss was raised about Kevorkian's predations until he participated in the death of a man, despite his having previously "helped" a dozen women to their deaths. One hopes the hue and cry that erupted after the first death of a man was a coincidence.

Yet some patients do wish to define when the end of the line has come. And many will seek provider involvement. As in the case of Elizabeth Bouvia, they may even seek to force providers to help them commit suicide. Most of these patients will be women.

I strongly suggest that all providers, but especially those in dedicated women's programs, start thinking about how they would handle such a request.

Are we dealing in myth and stereotype to promote women's wishes? Are women healthcare professionals better—just because they are women? As more women become administrators and physicians, new questions about the social ethics of women's care arise. American healthcare, despite its essentially female nature and history, is still controlled by men. That is not going to be the case in 20 years, but it is the case now. That means an uphill fight for an equal shake for women in healthcare leadership.

It also means that we must be cautious about creating the image that all women doctors are good doctors, just because they are women. Are we giving them a free ride because baby boomer women seem to prefer them, and because most of them are young and suit the culture of our programs? I think the different attitudes often exhibited by women physicians have far more to do with the fact that most of them are under 40 than with their gender; we should not misinterpret their style as being simply the result of their sex.

More generally, the segregation of women in women's healthcare programs may not, in the long run, prove to be the best way to go. Segregating the sexes in the guise of providing women with appropriate care is a thorny issue, and one on which I have not made up my mind. But I don't think we should simply accept it without continuing reassessment.

Is the growing popularity of denying services to the elderly tied to the fact that most of them are female? We hear a lot of talk about rationing of care these days, but there is an aspect of rationing that has not been acknowledged very often. The vast majority of the elderly, especially the advanced elderly, are women—and their proportion is growing. More than 70 percent of the elderly over 85 are women. And elderly women are simply devalued.

I used to write obituaries for a living, and to this day I read the obituary pages. They concern men ten times more often than women. Is that because women don't die? No, it's due to the fact that most women are not considered noteworthy. Ever read an obituary that says, "Hattie Francis, 85, former sharecropper, who raised ten children who all went to college, died today in Pascagoula . . ."?

Rationing of healthcare, at this point in its development, has too often become a synonym for robbing the helpless and poor to keep the wealthy comfortable. Advocates for women should not support denying necessary services to people just because they are little old ladies. We'll be there soon enough ourselves.

Are the poor being treated? If you hang out a shingle that says you are providing healthcare to women, the ethics of language, of commitment, and of personal morality dictate that you must mean more by that than "a program of selected services for well-heeled, lavishly insured baby-boomer white women who aren't very sick." There is a universe of need out there.

The majority of the uninsured poor are women and children. The same is true of those "covered" by Medicaid. Often, they cannot get care; if they do, it is often too late and it is paid for with constant fear and loss of human dignity. This is an ironic juxtaposition with the sensitivity of our women's centers, and it raises obvious moral questions—questions that go far beyond issues of financing.

Those who call themselves women's healthcare professionals who are not actively—passionately—involved in the fight for universal access are lying to themselves about what they do for a living. Those in need are not defined as those who pass the social or financial test of acceptability in a given program. Need is where we find it.

We find it in the 35 million people living in poverty, again, most of them women and children. In the hundreds of thousands of unmarried teenage mothers. In the thousands of AIDS patients who are women. In the women increasingly being diagnosed with genetic defects, and promptly kicked out of the insurance system, such as the pregnant woman who was found to have the gene for cystic fibrosis and then informed that her employer would not cover her unless she had an abortion.

We find it in the addicted women who are castigated as criminals and excluded, if pregnant, from most drug treatment programs, while football players and other celebrities enter and leave these programs with the ease of people using the subway.

We find need in the millions of women suffering from severe mental illness, who are not wanted by the boutique psychiatric facilities or the mainstream healthcare system, and who too often find their ultimate answer in murder or suicide. In the battered women whose terror-filled existence, given the shortage of counseling and shelter, too often fulfills the old definition of the life of the poor: nasty, brutish, and short.

Do something! So I close with a plea that you do something for the excluded women. Start a WIC (Women, Infants, and Children) program, as many hospitals have done. Start accepting Medicaid patients—AFDC and long-term care alike. Start a community program to reduce infant mortality. Link up with shelters for battered women and programs for addicted women. Lobby for drug treatment programs to accept addicted pregnant women.

Work on a comprehensive, community-based program for Alzheimer's patients, who are statistically more likely to be women. Link up with long-term care programs for frail women with no immediate family. Start up a foster grandparents' program.

Thousands of women endured disdain and humiliation, struggled, suffered, and sometimes died to create what is emerging now as a society in which women are seen as valuable, individual, and worthwhile. Our best way to honor their legacy is to extend that emerging tolerance to those who are still cast aside.

And even though we cannot be all things to all women in practice, we can represent all women in spirit—including the poverty-stricken, the old and frail, the crippled, the syphilitic, the mad, the hopeless, and the different. If we do not stand up for them, who will?

And if healthcare providers, who represent the last and best hope of so many of them, fail them instead, then who is it we seek to serve?

Marya Mannes, an American writer, said it all: "Women are repeatedly accused of taking things personally. I cannot see any other honest way of taking them." We should take the failures of our healthcare system in terms of women very personally—and we should do something about them.

* * * * * * *

Women's Wishes: "Unreflective, Immature"

How are women patients' wishes treated with regard to terminating treatment? This concern was raised in an article by Steven H. Miles, MD, and Allison August in the Summer 1990 issue of Law, Medicine, and Healthcare ("Courts, Gender, and `the Right to Die'"). The authors surveyed how the courts treat male and female patient-plaintiffs in terms of decisions to terminate treatment.

The results are depressing. First, they found, the courts view men's wishes as "rational" and women's wishes as "unreflective, emotional, or immature." Thus, not surprisingly, evidence is interpreted differently for men and women. Men who are on life support are viewed as being subject to assault; women are viewed as "vulnerable to medical neglect."

Studying all appellate cases over 14 years involving patients' rights with respect to termination of life support, Miles and August found that male claimants were generally judged in terms of their personal wishes and rights, whereas female claimants were judged in terms of their relationship to society and what society wanted to do with them or wanted them to do.

Women's healthcare professionals hold a special responsibility to protect their patients against a court system that may well view them as tools of social policy, rather than as individuals.

This is particularly an issue for an aging population of women. The force of demographics, which fueled the creation of many women's centers and programs, is now guaranteeing that most aged, frail, and potentially incompetent patients will be women living alone. In the absence of clear and convincing evidence of their wishes, they can be subjected to existence-prolonging technology for very dubious reasons. It is therefore incumbent upon those who care for them to see that each of them has a living will and preferably a durable power of attorney.

We must protect all patients from technological, political, and ideological excess; but women are at special risk. In the words of California physician Valerie Berry in her lovely poem, "Intensive Care":

> Your men are gone.
> Father, husband, sons who waltzed with you
> Have faded into the wallpaper roses.
> There is no one to lead you in this last number.
> We are two girls in white left to learn
> the final steps together.

It has always come down to this:

Women teaching women how to live.

(From *"Intensive Care,"* by *Valerie Berry*, MD, published in the *Western Journal of Medicine*, December 1988, page 717)

. . . .

This article is based on a presentation made to the National Association of Women's Health Professionals in 1990.

Freedom of Choice

March 1994

*This is the second in an occasional series of columns
examining the ethics side of healthcare reform.
The first, "A Matter of Principle," appeared in
the September 1992 issue.*

"Fighting words" are statements that stir emotions so deeply
that people get violent over them. And few phrases cut to
the heart of the American psyche like those three little words, "freedom of choice." They represent a principle, a form of political and
social organization, and a way of life.

Freedom of choice is a powerful concept. We believe in it profoundly. We believe in it even when it doesn't seem to make much
sense. In the face of the deadly privation occurring in Bosnia,
Somalia, Angola, and other suffering places, for example, I sometimes wonder if it is really necessary for Americans to have a
choice of 42 different kinds of facial tissue. Our tears don't care
what they get sopped up with, and there are undoubtedly better
uses for those resources.

In trying to answer my question, I have to remind myself that it
may not be *economically* necessary to have all those competing
brands of tissue, but it is *culturally* necessary. We want to have a
choice. We want options.

So it's not surprising that if we take the powerful phrase "freedom of choice" and inject it into the very emotional and personal world of healthcare reform, more than a few fights result. And it is entirely possible that the battles over this concept will be among the most emotional, fervent, and intellectually dishonest fights in the reform debate.

There is certainly an issue here. In the first place, social legislation—or any other kind of legislation—almost always involves constraining someone's freedom to do something. We don't want people to run red lights or drive 150 miles an hour or machine-gun people in shopping malls. We pass laws to prevent and punish such activity.

At the same time we enthusiastically sell—and buy—cars that can grossly exceed the speed limit and automatic weapons that would do most terrorists proud. There is an inherent tension in supporting governments and laws that constrain us, but we have decided (most of us, anyway) that it beats the alternative.

Healthcare reform is no different. There are all kinds of potential restrictions: on the number of plans available, on the amount of money to be spent, on how services are used and offered, on providers' options, on patients' options, on payers' options. Some proposals would get rid of private payers; others would essentially banish fee-for-service medicine. No matter what the plan, there will be limits on freedom.

But we live with such limits now in healthcare; few of us can choose any insurer we want, who will pay any provider we pick for whatever service we use, regardless of appropriateness, quality, or price. Reform will not change that; there will still be constraints on freedom. But it will be a case of changing the type of constraint, rather than introducing constraints for the first time.

There is more to the issue than that. Most major players in reform are seeking to be seen as the champions of preserving freedom of choice. Everyone from the commercial insurance lobby to organized medicine wants to be associated with the concept. In public statements, press releases, advertisements, speeches, and writings, each entity claims that higher ground.

Which Choice?

But what do they mean by freedom of choice? What is it that these combatants are claiming to want to preserve? I think we are, in fact, debating four issues: choice of insurer, choice of type of insurer, choice of physician, and retention of physician. In each case, the situation—and the probable outcome—is different.

1. Choice of insurer. The commercial carriers, especially those represented by the Health Insurance Association of America, have sought to use this issue to defeat the Clinton plan, by running television and print ads suggesting that there will be no freedom of choice of insurer under managed competition.

Under "pure" managed competition (if there is such a thing), there would certainly be fewer insurance plans than there are now. That is because under pure managed competition, the purchasing cooperatives or health alliances or whatever the heck they're being called this week are only supposed to contract with a very few plans. The whole idea is to force insurers and providers into Darwinian combat that only some would survive.

But "pure" managed competition is not what the reformers are talking about. Except for some of the single-payer advocates, most politicians are unwilling to partially or totally destroy the commercial insurance industry. So the proposals that are based on managed competition tend to have provisions stating that an alliance must sign up any plan that meets its criteria.

Besides, commercial insurers are turning out to be the Steven Seagal of healthcare: They're hard to kill. The state of Vermont, for example, passed reform legislation that was designed in part to reduce the number of insurers in the state. The legislation included stringent restrictions on insurance marketing and underwriting, and many pundits expected most of the commercial carriers to leave town. Nonetheless, there are still many commercial insurers in Vermont.

Needless to say, freedom of choice of insurer is a critically important issue for insurers. But is it so critical to the public? When you get right down to it, most people don't have a choice of insurer now. The Kaiser/Commonwealth Fund Health Insurance Survey, conducted in late 1993 by Louis Harris and Associates, found this to be the case. Of Americans surveyed, 44 percent of those who have coverage through an employer or union have a choice of only one plan, and 57 percent of those employed in smaller firms are offered only one plan.

For the most part, a choice of dozens of different plans is available only to federal employees and a few other groups. Theoretically, individuals who are seeking coverage on their own should have a much wider choice than those who must accept their employers' selection. But few insurers have much, if any, interest in the individual market; many have gotten out of it entirely, and others have limited enrollment or closed it to new members.

Ironically, despite the commercial insurers' howls, most reform proposals would increase the individual's choice of insurer. And I don't think most Americans have warm and fuzzy feelings about "their" insurance companies, so I don't see this as a particularly emotional issue for anyone except insurers.

2. Choice of type of insurance. Will indemnity insurance and fee-for-service payment survive reform? Or will managed care and capitated payment take over? This is an issue for providers and insurers who don't like managed care or who don't think they would do well in an environment dominated by managed care.

I wouldn't stay up late worrying about it. This is America, the land of 42 kinds of facial tissue. Under most reform proposals, fee-for-service healthcare and indemnity insurance would survive—albeit with a stiff premium, which will make it more of a boutique activity than a dominant model.

But it's a bit late to be bringing this up. A KPMG Peat Marwick survey of employee health benefits in late 1993 found that more than 95 percent of the people who have coverage through employment are already in some form of managed care—some form of HMO, some form of PPO, or some type of "managed indemnity."

The market has shifted. This battle is pretty much over, and managed care has won, at least for the time being.

That is not to say there are not battles ahead. There are many kinds of managed care, and the different models will slug it out in coming years. That will be a change from the situation that has prevailed in most places until now, which was competition between managed care and fee-for-service indemnity models.

Now we will be asking different questions. Can managed care plans pay on a fee-for-service basis and compete successfully? (Probably not.) Do closed-panel HMOs like Kaiser or Humana offer better quality and higher efficiency? (That tends to be the prevailing wisdom.) Will new models crop up that differ from traditional HMO structures? (They are already doing so; indeed, we could end up with as many types of managed care as we have of facial tissue.)

Also, it is not enough to say that the public has accepted the management of its healthcare. It has, but the acceptance has not always been voluntary. And there is some wariness among those who have never belonged to an HMO: The Kaiser/Commonwealth Survey found that 52 percent of non-HMO members express concern about being required to join one. And people are wary of cheap plans: The survey also revealed that only 30 percent of those who have a choice pick the least expensive plan offered.

But that is not a core middle-class issue. Cheap, lowball HMOs tend to be the province of Medicaid beneficiaries and other powerless populations who have little or no choice in the matter. The quality of the plans that they and previously uninsured low-income people may end up being forced to join is a very serious issue.

There is a dismal history in this country of poor people's HMOs that have been scandal-ridden, shoddy, and corrupt. Without proper safeguards, that history could be repeated in the future, especially in those states (Oregon, Tennessee, Florida, and others) where forced enrollment of Medicaid clients in HMOs is being used as a cost-containment mechanism. As I have often said, I think good managed care is a superior form of health service structure, especially for vulnerable patients; but not all managed care is good.

Thus, even if it is not a matter of great concern to the rich and powerful (most of whom do not belong to HMOs, good or bad), freedom of choice of type of plan will be a matter of ethical concern as long as powerless, vulnerable people are forced into lowball, insufficiently monitored managed care plans from which they cannot escape.

3. Choice of physician. The issue of freedom of choice of physician is much more substantive for patients than arcane debates over insurance structure. But it is really two issues.

The first issue—freedom of choice of provider—does matter to people. The Kaiser survey showed that 50 percent of Americans find it unacceptable to limit choice of surgeons, 49 percent object to limited choice of specialists, 40 percent object to limited choice of generalist physicians, and 38 percent object to limited choice of pediatrician.

Interestingly, 48 percent object to limited choice of hospitals, despite the fact that relatively few Americans under 65 years old have much say about which hospital they use. I ascribe this response to the visceral reaction many of us have when we are told our choice of anything is to be constrained—even if it's something we have never used and don't want to use.

But I don't think the right to pick any doctor you want is the basic issue. We have to find new physicians all the time. We leave town. The doctor leaves town. One or the other moves to a new neighborhood. Our primary care relationships change frequently as physicians join or leave HMOs. The kids grow up and don't need a pediatrician anymore. Your parents age and they need a gerontologist.

In a mobile society, people need to find new doctors on a regular basis. And most people don't choose their specialists; they generally use the one to whom they are referred by another physician.

4. Retention of physician. This debate is not about *choice* of physician so much as it is about *retention* of physician. People don't want ongoing relationships disrupted when they don't have to be. In survey after survey, study after study, that's what the real public concern turns out to be. Certainly, if a physician moves or dies, we have no choice about seeking a new one, but we don't want to be forced by policy or payer to leave a trusted doctor.

The level of concern over this is not uniform; it is much more serious for certain people, especially older patients. Why do so few Medicare patients join HMOs, despite 20 years of efforts to cajole them into doing so? Because they don't want to end long-term relationships with physicians. This is a special issue for older people because Medicare patients use a great deal of healthcare. Teenagers, on the other hand, change doctors the way most people change socks.

One interesting study by Shoshanna Sofaer and Margo-Lea Hurwicz (*Medical Care*, September 1993) found, for example, that when physicians in a medical group left an HMO and joined another one, 60 percent of their Medicare patients followed the doctors.

So of these four debates over freedom of choice, the one about retaining a physician with whom you have had a long relationship is the one most likely to see heavy public involvement. The Clinton plan and other managed competition schemes acknowledge this; their backers have stated repeatedly that you can keep your physicians—as long as they sign up with the same plan you join.

Think about that. It means that insurance companies, HMOs, and health alliances, who decide which physicians they accept, will determine whether you can, in fact, stick with your doctor. When the public figures that out, it may be less than enchanted with the idea. At that point, you may see growing support for a single-payer plan, which provides no choice of payer—but full choice of provider.

The Limits of Choice

There are two other points we should keep in mind. The first is that for approximately 50 million people, the primary source of care is their friendly neighborhood emergency department. I don't think many of them are going to be frantic about whether they will be able to retain their ER or not. For a large segment of the population, the argument about retention of physician is meaningless, because they don't have one to retain.

The other point is that the people of the United States, even as they pick and choose among facial tissues, do not have an unlimited appetite for making choices. Economists and policy wonks are dying to unload outcomes data and comparative plan data and price data onto the public, in order to foster "more informed consumer choices." But when people are healthy, they are not particularly interested in healthcare data—especially in the incomprehensible form in which we offer them.

And when people are sick or injured, often their choices are made for them by others. After being hit by a truck, one does not lie in the ambulance comparing outcomes data in order to decide which trauma center to use.

And how many of us really want to read pitches from 35 different plans and decide among them? The federal employee health benefits program, which is supposed to be a model of managed competition, offers many insurance choices. Yet in 1993, 41 percent of its members still picked Blue Cross and Blue Shield.

As the ice cream maker Howard Johnson once lamented, "I've spent my entire life developing ice cream flavors, and most people still say, 'I'll take vanilla.'" In the end, given a wide range of choices, people often choose what's familiar.

None of this should be interpreted to mean that I do not think choice is a valid issue in reform; far from it. Indeed, I have grumped about my HMO's restrictions on my options on more than one occasion, and I have many friends who, facing serious illness in their families, want to head off to the Mayo Clinic or to Beth Israel Hospital in Boston, only to find that their insurance does not allow it.

One might envy Medicare patients, who can usually still make such choices; the constraints on freedom in the Medicare program fall far more heavily on providers than on patients. That is the tradeoff under single-payer programs like Medicare. We have yet to see whose freedom will be compromised most by reform. But it's safe to say that it will be one heck of a fight.

• • • • • • •

This column is based on remarks presented at an Estes Park Institute conference in Naples, Florida, December 1993.

Helplessness and Goodness

May 1994

"There goes the neighborhood." That was my ironic joke to myself on January 17 of this year, as I watched parts of the San Fernando Valley—where I lived as a child—crumble and burn in the wake of the Northridge earthquake. I called a dear friend from childhood, who had lived a block away. She said, "It's like losing your history."

Most of my family members live in or near the Valley, but I couldn't get through by phone to find out if they were alive or dead. (All of them suffered damage to their homes and/or possessions and one relative was injured, but they all survived.) I called and called, but it was to no avail—as was the case for millions of others in the same boat.

It was 25 degrees below zero in Chicago, where I live, so life was paralyzed on my end of things as well. My car did not want to go anywhere, the wind-chill factor was minus-60 degrees, and the authorities were warning people not to go outside.

I felt helpless, with no control whatsoever over the events affecting me. So I sat there for two days and watched the earthquake's aftermath on television.

And I learned something—or, rather, was reminded of something.

First came that horrible television image of the fallen building with the words "Kaiser Permanente" on the side. "Oh, my God, a hospital's down." No, it was a clinic and administration building; no one was inside when the quake hit.

Then the camera panned from the Kaiser facility to the nearby Granada Hills Community Hospital parking lot, where, with the earth still quivering, hundreds of people were being triaged and cared for by hospital staff. The television news crew (with the all-too-common lack of sense for which the profession is becoming known) barged into the hospital to get pictures of the injured. The hospital staff, up to their behinds in alligators, were still quite courteous in asking the crew to leave.

When We Are Called . . .

At that point, two ideas came to me. The first was that the news crew was hardly short of things to broadcast. At that time, there were dreadful fires in several locations, three major freeways were down, homes were sliding down mountainsides, and an entire apartment complex had imploded on itself, killing many of its residents while they slept.

But the news people focused on the hospitals. Why? Because they wanted to show that something was working, that the world had not gone completely awry. Because, even if they were not aware of it, they wanted comfort, too.

When things start going very, very badly, we as a society turn to three sources of comfort: police, fire departments, and the health-care system.

My simultaneous second thought was one of envy, strangely enough. There I sat, unable to do anything about all the fears that were assailing me, but the nurses, physicians, technicians, administrators, security people, and others at those Los Angeles hospitals *could* do something. And they were doing it. I was reminded, from my own experience of working in low-level jobs in several hospitals, that one of the opportunities healthcare gives us is the chance to do something when just about everyone else is helpless.

It is more than that. It is that people, when they are helpless, either in the grip of an individual disease or of a community disaster, whether they are injured patients or frightened loved ones or reporters trying to cover a story, turn instinctively to healthcare providers for help.

Being empowered to act when few others can do so is an opportunity and a responsibility at the same time. It presents us with the highest of ethical imperatives: When we are called, we have to go.

What is so stunning about the power of that ethic is that when calamity hits, healthcare people rarely have to be reminded of their responsibility.

A Few Stories

There will be many stories and articles and books and movies about the Los Angeles earthquake (I'm sure the television networks are already in production with their efforts). There have been or will be words and film and tape about the Loma Prieta quake in San Francisco, Hurricane Andrew, Hurricane Iniki, and the Mississippi River floods.

One hopes that healthcare folk will receive proper recognition. I'm sure many people have better stories than the ones I have heard, but to illustrate how healthcare folks respond to threats to their neighbors, let me cite a few:

- A group of physicians from the University of California-Irvine Medical Center in Orange County, more than 50 miles away from Northridge, picked their way through fallen freeways and shaking ground to help out their colleagues at hospitals near the epicenter.

- Nearly 100 healthcare professionals—including people who work in security and central supply—volunteered to fly from other islands in Hawaii to help providers on the devastated island of Kauai after Hurricane Iniki, knowing full well they were going into a situation with little food or water and virtually no shelter, during rainy season.

- Physicians from Memorial Hospital in Hollywood, Florida, the day after Hurricane Andrew hit, realized that all the pharmacies were gone in the Homestead area, thus threatening the health of patients dependent on insulin, anti-hypertensive drugs, and other medications. They filled a van with pharmaceuticals and prescription pads, and went into the devastation to provide free care and drugs to the chronically ill.

- The staff of Saint John's Hospital and Medical Center in Santa Monica evacuated pregnant women, mothers, and infants shortly after the Northridge quake from a building that could have fallen on them at any time; no one suffered so much as a scratch.

- So many healthcare folk, in these disasters and many others, either chose to go to the hospital or clinic immediately (when there was no warning), or volunteered to stay extra shifts (in those instances when there was some warning)—often not even knowing if they had a home to return to. In the case of Iniki, they knew without checking that they had probably lost everything they owned. And when the reporters asked, "How are things at home?," they replied, nonchalantly, "I don't know; I haven't been home since this happened."

Ten days after the earthquake, I found myself on the island of Molokai in Hawaii, visiting the sites where Father Damien DeVeuster

(1840-1889) spent 17 years caring for the patients with Hansen's disease (then known as leprosy) who had been exiled by law to the Kalaupapa peninsula, surrounded on two sides by ocean and on the third by 3,000-foot-high cliffs. It was a one-way trip for them, as it was for Damien; he died there of the disease that afflicted his parishioners.

Our guide on that day was Richard Marks, a third-generation Molokai exile; he continues to live in Kalaupapa, although the quarantine order was lifted in 1969. As we sat in Saint Philomena's Church, much of which Father Damien built with his own hands, Marks made a telling comment: "Damien wasn't a doctor; he couldn't do anything about the people's disease. But he could take care of them, change their bandages, help them die as Christians."

In Damien's time, even doctors could not do anything about Hansen's disease. But the Belgian farm boy who had become a priest was able to act in the face of helpless doctors and helpless patients alike: He cared. He fought for resources for his sick brethren, loved them, washed their bodies, bandaged their sores, and healed their souls. Even when nothing clinical could be done, he was able to do something equally important: He protected them from the curse of helplessness.

Are Healthcare People Unusually Good?

All these are acts of healthcare heroism, in one way or another. So one must ask: Do people go into healthcare to be heroes? I doubt it. One cannot predict with certainty that one will be called on to be heroic, and few of us know how we would react if the call came.

Are people in healthcare inordinately altruistic? I don't know. Certainly, most healthcare folk are paid for what they do (although the level of volunteerism in healthcare exceeds that of most other sectors of American life). But they do seem, consistently, to have a capacity for self-sacrifice when the chips are down.

Then are healthcare people unusually good? I realize that it is unfashionable to use a term such as "goodness," but if I learned anything from my two helpless days watching the earthquake, it is that if we believe there is evil in this world, then we should believe that there is goodness here as well. I don't know if we all possess equal amounts of good and evil, or whether these capacities are unevenly distributed in each of us (I suspect the latter, but I will leave the debate to the theologians, who have been discussing the subject for some 20 centuries).

What I do know is that calamity—individual or societal—produces two interlocking needs in our society: on the one side, a need for help, for healing, and for security, and on the other side, a need to provide help, healing, and security. Those two needs come together in healthcare.

Healthcare folk are not unique in having the chance to be good; certainly the inordinate sacrifices of those who saved Jews, Gypsies, Poles, and others from the Nazis were the highest possible examples of goodness. Indeed, I do not know how else to explain the Raoul Wallenbergs and Oskar Schindlers of this world except to say that goodness is a mystery that should be acknowledged, respected, and encouraged, even though we may not understand it.

Nonetheless, people in healthcare are given the opportunity to act when others cannot, on a more regular basis than just about anyone other than police officers and firefighters. So it may be that they are not necessarily exceptionally good, but that they have the chance to do good more than most people do.

The question is, can we live our lives on this principle? Can we be expected to give our all on a daily basis? Madeline Bohman, when she was CEO of Bellevue Hospital Center in New York City, once said, "This place operates beautifully during a disaster. I just wish I could get the mail delivered more quickly on an average day."

I don't think we can live with incredibly high levels of adrenaline surging through our systems constantly. If we did, we wouldn't last very long. (This does not explain the life of emergency department professionals, but they are a wondrous and separate breed unto themselves.)

But we can certainly keep in the back of our minds that we have this singular opportunity—to answer helplessness with goodness—and that few others are so graced.

A Train from Boston

On December 6, 1917, in the narrows between Halifax and Dartmouth, Nova Scotia, an overloaded ammunition ship, the *Mont Blanc*, collided with another ship, caught fire, and exploded.

The blast was the worst man-made explosion in recorded history prior to Hiroshima. It leveled a square mile of Halifax, killed at least 2,000 people, set much of the remaining town on fire, and drove shards of glass into the eyes of hundreds of survivors. The suffering was so awful that one of the physicians on the scene hanged himself a short time later.

One of the worst blizzards in Nova Scotia history hit the next day, leaving rescuers to work in waist-high snow and slush.

Within hours, into that horror came a train from Boston carrying medical supplies, in an effort said to have been spearheaded by the Massachusetts Eye and Ear Hospital. The next day a second train arrived from Boston, fighting its way through the blizzard, carrying enough equipment for a 500-bed hospital as well as 25 physicians, two obstetricians, 68 nurses, and eight orderlies. To this day, the city of Halifax sends the city of Boston a pine tree at Christmas every year in remembrance.

With all the provider-bashing that is going on, it is important to remember that people—even economists—turn to healthcare providers when they are afraid or in trouble. It is our responsibility to return that trust with goodness.

And far more often than not, we do. For that, a pine tree to all: It is richly deserved.

How We Keep Score

July 1994

Fifteen years ago, one of the big issues in healthcare was the growth of for-profit healthcare enterprises and what their effect on the healthcare system might be. The possibility of their having a negative influence was raised by the then-editor of the *New England Journal of Medicine*, Arnold Relman, MD, in his classic essay, "The Medical-Industrial Complex," published in that journal on October 23, 1980. He questioned the values and practices of proprietary firms ranging from hospital chains to kidney dialysis services.

Interestingly, Relman did not include physicians, despite the fact that either as practitioners or as entrepreneurs in larger efforts, they generally fall into the for-profit category. His focus was on corporate activity.

There were predictions, back then, that for-profit chains would soon dominate the hospital field, and that voluntary providers should fear for their lives. That did not come to pass, however, and the controversy died down.

Renewed Debate

The debate has been reinvigorated in recent years, because of several events. One development was rapid growth in physician self-referral—that is, a physician sending patients to healthcare services in which he or she has a financial interest. Revelations of possible improprieties led, in fairly short order, to federal and state legislation limiting the practice.

A second factor has been wider public knowledge of the income of physicians and other healthcare professionals, especially hospital executives. Indeed, it has become common practice in some cities (Boston and Omaha, for two) for newspapers to publish hospital CEOs' salaries.

Among others whose annual income has become a matter of public record are the leaders of healthcare suppliers such as U.S. Surgical and Medco Containment, and the heads of for-profit chains—Thomas Frist, Jr., MD, chairman and CEO of HCA, received $127 million in compensation in 1992, raising more than a few eyebrows. A Massachusetts HMO that was going bankrupt paid its five top executives $1.2 million in 1991.

The emergence of Columbia Healthcare Corporation, which acquired the Galen and HCA hospital firms, has lent fuel to the fire. Columbia owns approximately 195 hospitals, with more on the way. It is dominant in some markets, such as south Florida, and its high-profile CEO, Richard Scott, does not calm people's nerves with remarks like "We . . . have the goal of owning 100 percent of the markets" where his firm has a presence. Scott's personal Columbia stock holdings are said to be worth $266.7 million.

Remember when Lee Iacocca was pilloried in the press for accepting his $20 million salary while Chrysler was struggling? His salary was 7 percent of Scott's reported worth.

A third factor sparking the discussion is the growth of proprietary enterprise in healthcare across the board. For-profit insurers remain big players; nearly 100 million Americans are covered by these firms. Although nonprofit Blue Cross and Blue Shield remains the largest insurer, it is an open secret that a debate is raging among its member plans about the desire of some to convert to for-profit status (some say that California Blue Cross has essentially done so).

Among HMOs, 67.4 percent are proprietary, with 20.4 million members. And, of course, most healthcare suppliers are proprietary;

the profits and pricing policies of pharmaceutical firms have been a major bone of policy contention for years.

Even a casual survey of providers finds a significant for-profit presence there as well. Among nongovernment community hospitals, 14 percent were proprietary in 1992, as were 11 percent of hospital beds; that number is likely to be higher because of Columbia acquisitions. Of nursing homes, 73 percent are for-profit, as are 71 percent of the beds.

In fact, with the exception of hospitals, for-profit firms and/or activities dominate all major provider sectors: medicine, nursing homes, group practices, HMOs, home healthcare, and others. And all this happened after the for-profit "scare" was said to be a false alarm.

This is to say nothing of the fact that many hospitals, HMOs, and other providers are heavily indebted to for-profit banks and other lenders from whom they have borrowed billions, and who thus could have a say in how the provider conducts business.

Is this cause for panic? Does for-profit activity, as Dr. Relman suggested, pose a grave threat to the mission, ethics, and performance of healthcare entities? Several issues are worth pondering.

Ownership or Behavior?

Is for-profit activity the same as for-profit ownership? I don't think so; indeed, there is a critical distinction.

For years, nonprofit hospitals condemned for-profits as though being a proprietary entity, in itself, constituted a sin. Or, perhaps, as though being a voluntary nonprofit entity, in itself, constituted moral superiority.

Neither perception is accurate. Many proprietary firms have modest profit margins, provide a great deal of community service, support charitable foundations, and engage in community benefit activities. They also provide income (through stock dividends) to many other Americans, and they pay at least some taxes.

In fact, Richard Scott has been quoted as saying that "non-taxpaying hospitals shouldn't be in business. They're not good corporate citizens." (Until recently, of course, Columbia was headquartered in Texas, which has no personal or corporate income tax. But we'll discuss that another time.)

Some nonprofits, on the other hand, have not exactly been model charities. Consider the hospital with $100 million in the bank that announced it "could not afford" to provide emergency services to the uninsured poor. Another voluntary hospital had a "margin" so high, and provided so little charity care, that the state in which it was located passed a law requiring hospitals to provide a minimum amount of indigent care. Some voluntary hospitals were just as guilty as for-profits of "dumping" indigent patients, a practice so dangerous that eventually state and federal law banned it.

The issue is not ownership; the issue is behavior.

That said, there are certain reasons for being concerned about investor-owned providers. These have to do with inherent conflicts of interest, not necessarily with behavior.

The first potential problem is that the trustees of a publicly held for-profit organization have a primary legal, fiduciary, and ethical duty to enhance profit for stockholders—which is as it should be. Unfortunately, this offers the possibility of patient or public welfare taking a back seat when the two are in conflict.

Second, the profits that pour into corporate bottom lines and shareholders' pockets leave healthcare and don't come back. When 44 percent of all healthcare expenditures come from taxes (and a much higher percentage of the funds that go to hospitals, nursing homes, and physicians are public monies), it is a legitimate point of ethical debate as to whether payments to shareholders are the best use of those profits—especially in a nation with 38 million uninsured people, where babies die of measles.

It is for these two reasons that I have doubts about the appropriateness of for-profit dominance of healthcare delivery.

Hospitals Are Different

Other questions that do not involve ownership are also worth asking. One is why hospitals, alone among providers, have remained predominantly nonprofit. Is there something about them that makes them different?

Yes, there is: The public thinks they are different. Just about everyone uses a hospital at one time or another, often in exigency. These are the places where we are born and often where we die, where we bleed, where we hope to heal. That is probably why the vast majority of hospitals have deep roots in the communities where they are located.

The history of hospitals is full of tales of people scrounging money, mortgaging homes, holding bake sales, begging and borrowing, and sometimes constructing hospitals with their own hands, because this was something they wanted their communities to have. They certainly did not think of their hospitals in terms of what financial rewards they would yield.

Other hospitals were the product of religious faith, founded by members of religious orders and congregations who often underwent major hardships in order to realize their dream.

Among organizational providers, hospitals are the oldest, are used by more people, have stronger community roots, and are more likely to be needed in an emergency. It is not surprising that the people who created them did not think of them in terms of profit.

But the public's perception has changed. Now it links hospitals and profit. A 1991 study found that 47 percent of the public thought their local hospitals were for-profit; 50 percent thought hospitals should be required to pay property taxes.

It is likely that this misperception developed in the Seventies and Eighties, when voluntary hospitals became enamored of business language and cut-throat competition. The explosive growth of proprietary hospitals and other services provided competition, but it also provided a model. Nonprofits somehow thought they could compete aggressively, select patients on the basis of income and coverage, duplicate services, develop for-profit subsidiaries left and right, and act just like proprietary entities—and no one would notice.

They were wrong. And the question now is what kind of relationship the public wants to have with them. That relationship will, in large measure, govern the nature of the regulatory environment in which hospitals operate in the future.

This is, of course, related to the delicate issue of tax status. Most of the activities pursued by voluntary hospitals in order to differentiate themselves from for-profit institutions and organizations have been tied to repeated threats to voluntary hospitals' tax-exempt status.

Ever since 1969, when the Internal Revenue Service rescinded its requirement that a nonprofit hospital provide indigent care and replaced it with a vague requirement for community service, hospitals have been trying to decide what that means, at least in terms of retaining tax-exempt status. The question has not yet been answered definitively, either by hospitals or government.

However, it seems to me that retention of tax status is a weak reason for identifying oneself as a voluntary organization. It is, in fact, a rather cynical quest: an effort to keep the tax man away while, in some cases, getting away with as little charitable service and community benefit as possible. Through such means, a redundant, poor-quality provider could well retain its tax status, but the ethical choice would probably be for it to close its doors.

This gets back to the idea that nonprofit status, all by itself, makes an organization morally superior; it does nothing of the kind. Tax status should be a reflection of performance. Being tax-exempt is simply not automatically equivalent to being a community-oriented, charitable institution or organization.

Enough Is Enough

A related issue is that of personal profit. Egregious personal self-inurement in healthcare is not ethically defensible, whether it occurs in the for-profit or the nonprofit sector. To the degree that we allow it, it taints us all.

In 1992, for example, a California neurologist made national headlines after he was told by his accountant that he needed to spend $10,000 in order to get a tax break. He went to the Super Bowl in Minneapolis-St. Paul, paid $1,550 a ticket for himself and three physician companions, rented a Rolls-Royce, and told a reporter that he "plays hard." He also wrote it all off, or at least tried to, by claiming that he and his pals talked about neurology at half-time.

When physicians grumble about public hostility to them and their profession, when hospital and HMO executives are offended by publication of their salaries, when providers are hauled into congressional hearings and attacked, when laws and regulations reducing provider reimbursement are adopted, remember that it is the bad actors who are thought to represent all of us. Our weakest links are the ones that drag us all down.

When overcharging and corruption were revealed in the defense industry, an outraged public demanded action. Penalties were assessed, prosecutions conducted, contracts lost, firms barred from doing business with the federal government. And the once-sacrosanct defense sector became vulnerable to cost-cutting, base closings, and reductions in force that are still taking place.

With hospital occupancy at 63 percent, a glut of physicians, and profiteering at an all-time high, a similar onslaught against providers is hardly out of the question.

But even if the income is accrued through efficient business practices, is there a point at which enough is enough? Should one individual, no matter how talented, pull down $100 or $200 million in income derived from a human service that most of its customers are forced to use? Should we perhaps think about a special tax that would reclaim some part of these huge profits for the care of vulnerable populations, or some other means to recycle some of this money back into patient care?

Sure, Richard Scott's $267 million represents a measly .02 percent of the national total of $1.1 trillion spent on healthcare in a year. But it sure would immunize a lot of kids.

Profiteering is going to be even more of an issue under reform. Think about it. If costs are indeed going to be stabilized, then the window of opportunity for making obscene profits will close. That will likely spark a frenzy of activity from those who want to make a quick killing before it's too late. Coma recovery centers and liposuction clinics will spring up until the well runs dry. Quick-buck artists will find other ways to make themselves very rich.

Healthcare folk, if they have any sense, need to be on their guard against profiteering excess—on the part of competitors, hit-and-run entrepreneurs, and their own organizations.

Many providers recognize this and are examining their own actions more closely. Others couldn't care less. For still others, the issue presents a personal conflict. In a market-capital society such as ours, after all, profit is the mark of success. We do not celebrate the leaders of bankrupt organizations. Talk shows do not vie for guest appearances by corporate titans who went broke.

For many people, a good income—even better, a huge income—is validation of achievement. It means you won. As a character played by James Garner in the film *The Wheeler-Dealers* says, "The point of the game is not money. Money is just how we keep score."

Those pursuing a career in healthcare are not immune to the siren song of financial success. They have houses to pay off, children to put through school, retirements to think of. Like the rest of us, they also want to achieve professional success and, in many cases, leadership positions in their field. Healthcare can be an unforgiving employer; a fat bottom line is often a job ticket. Being seduced into putting profit first is an understandable reaction.

However, there is a great deal of middle ground between bankruptcy and the obscene piling up of profits. Rules can be developed to govern the conflicts inherent in allowing proprietary activities in an arena that the public sees as a voluntary public service.

The natural tension between for-profits and nonprofits can also be addressed in a civilized manner, rather than through repeated fits of name-calling. (I remember one Wall Street analyst praising HCA and insisting that Thomas Frist, Sr., MD, the firm's founder, had started the organization because "there were no decent hospitals in the South." That must have been news to Duke, Grady, Emory, Parkland, Jackson, and the many other great teaching centers and community hospitals of that region.)

Who's Minding the Store?

Princeton health economist Uwe Reinhardt once said that the venture capitalists came to healthcare because there was nowhere else in our economy for them to go. For decades now, their presence in this field has been a source of discomfort and debate.

I feel some of that discomfort, but that feeling is mild compared to the rage I have felt at the crimes committed by some organizations protected by the cloak of nonprofit status. In both cases, it is simply a matter of what standards of behavior should be expected in healthcare—and who should enforce them.

To the degree that we can make proper distinctions about behavior versus legal or tax status, for-profits and nonprofits should be able to coexist in healthcare, albeit with more than a little uneasiness. To the degree that we are able to clean up our act, rein in our excesses, and put our money to good use, we should be able to make—and enforce—our own rules about ethical profit-making and the future of the voluntary organization. To the degree that we ignore these issues, our missions will be defined for us by others.

Stanford medical economist Victor Fuchs, MD, has said that true cost containment in healthcare can be achieved only by paying one of three prices: providing fewer services, offering the same services with fewer resources, or lessening personal and organizational healthcare income. Given the opportunity, the public—the people who ultimately fund healthcare—would likely overwhelmingly vote for the third option. If we do not mind our store, and the money it makes, they might well be justified.

Losers

September 1994

This is the third in an occasional series of columns concerning ethics issues in healthcare reform. The first, "A Matter of Principle," and the second, "Freedom of Choice," appeared in the September 1992 and March 1994 issues, respectively.

Recently a noted healthcare economist was quoted as saying that competition in healthcare must be unfettered and unconstrained by government intervention, because if government is part of the process, it would likely be compelled to "indemnify the losers." Similarly, Stuart Altman, chairman of the Medicare Prospective Payment Assessment Commission, has pointed out that there is nothing wrong with a competitive approach to healthcare reform, but that "competition requires losers."

Indeed, despite all the rhetoric being bandied about by the major players in reform about the high motives they have for pursuing their particular causes, it is quite likely that much of the passion engendered by the reform debate is rooted in a fear of loss. Virtually everyone in the United States has something to lose in healthcare reform, even if we all also have much to gain.

Why do we talk about "winners" and "losers" in a public policy debate? The idea is to restructure healthcare financing and delivery, not to start a war, right?

Well, maybe so, but the fact is that when you start talking about restructuring, people tremble. And with good reason. The very term *restructuring,* in current American business, means lay-offs, downsizing, and elimination of unprofitable and inefficient holdings and practices. We've been restructuring the American military in the past few years, and among the visible results have been economic calamity in parts of California and other defense-dependent areas; people losing their jobs in both the military and the defense supply sector; the economic infrastructure of base towns being thrown into chaos—and government attempts to ameliorate the damage. One person's downsizing is another person's employment.

Little wonder, then, that the idea of reforming the U.S. health-care delivery system makes a lot of people who rely on that system for their livelihoods downright queasy.

Overbuilt and Bloated

They're right to worry. Our $1.1 trillion healthcare sector employs one of every 11 working Americans directly, with millions more dependent on it indirectly. Healthcare is a major factor in the stock market. American pharmaceuticals and medical technology are highly visible components of U.S. exports. Hospitals customarily rank among the top two or three biggest employers in town; in many rural areas, hospitals are the largest employers. In cities like Pittsburgh, Boston, and Honolulu, healthcare is among the largest business sectors in the area; in some, it is the largest.

Unfortunately, healthcare is also overbuilt and bloated. National hospital occupancy has ranged from 62 to 65 percent for years. In some badly overbuilt states such as California, it is much lower than that. As has been discussed for decades, the United States has more physicians per capita than any other nation, by far. We also have more of almost any other type of healthcare professional you can name, with the possible exception of nursing. More than 1,500 third-party payers foot the bill, which inevitably produces high administrative costs.

There is no way that reform, no matter how modest, will allow such excess to remain untouched.

In fact, this aspect of reform—restructuring of the delivery system—has already started. Mergers and alliances among providers are occurring everywhere. HMOs are buying each other. Hospitals are laying off workers of all kinds, from the dietary department to the administrative suite and even the department of nursing, long a sacrosanct exception. Physicians who pooh-poohed managed care and refused to sign contracts with HMOs are finding themselves frozen out of many markets.

It does not matter if federal reform is passed in any recognizable or meaningful form this year, or even if the leading reform states are able to implement the legislation they have passed. The shift to managed care, capitated payment, fewer and larger providers, and a leaner-and-meaner healthcare system has begun.

Who Are the Losers?

Who are the current and potential losers? On the provider side, hospitals with low occupancy and/or fewer paying patients. Hospitals providing trauma care, burn care, and other high-cost specialty services. Teaching hospitals. City and county hospitals.

People who work in endangered hospitals. Specialist physicians in glutted markets, especially those with high charges and little experience with managed care. Providers in thinly populated and/or low-income rural areas.

On the payer side, insurance brokers could be an endangered species if purchasing cooperatives that buy coverage directly become commonplace—and in several states, voluntary cooperatives are already up and running. Insurers whose main line of business is indemnity coverage. In some markets, insurers that have remained faithful to the ideals of community rating and acceptance of all applicants. HMOs that are only marginally competitive. HMOs that are likely takeover targets.

In the supply industry, downsizing will inevitably follow the downsizing of its customer base. Although some suppliers, such as the pharmaceutical houses, are already under the policy gun, it seems likely that manufacturers of big-ticket technology will find it a harder go as capitation takes hold. And new healthcare construction seems destined to continue to weaken.

On the patient side, in the absence of insurance reform and universal coverage (the absence of which seems just about certain), sicker patients, those with incurable illnesses, those with expensive illnesses, and those dependent on public programs (especially Medicaid) are also potential losers.

So, needless to say, are the poor. They could lose by being unattractive to HMOs; they could lose by being forcibly enrolled in managed care plans that earn their profits by denying appropriate access to care; and they could lose because the providers who have traditionally cared for them have become losers themselves. This is a particular concern in low-income rural and urban areas with few providers left, and is even more of a concern if the main source of care for the uninsured poor is a strapped public or religious-sponsored hospital that must compete for contracts in order to survive.

People Are Scared

It is hardly a surprise that we are starting to see some panic-stricken responses. State medical societies and other organized provider groups are pushing "any willing provider" legislation that requires managed care plans to contract with any provider willing to accept their payment rates. Needless to say, managed care plans oppose such laws, because they make it impossible to selectively contract with physicians and others.

There is frantic jockeying in Washington and in the state capitals by providers who want to make sure that their services are included in any statutorily defined basic benefit package. Others are demanding that they be deemed "essential community providers," with whom most or all payers must contract.

We are seeing the growth of physician unions, demands by physicians that they be exempted from antitrust laws so that they can bargain with payers in groups, and tough talk from labor unions representing healthcare workers.

People are scared. Despite their fears, it is unlikely that even the fiercest resistance will prevent the closing of hospitals, the consolidation of provider organizations, the reduction of physician and other provider incomes, the thinning out of the healthcare workforce, and the reconfiguration of American health insurance. Healthcare has been on a party for nearly 30 years, ever since Medicare and Medicaid opened the monetary floodgates in 1965. Now the morning after is looming.

And in all good conscience, it is difficult to argue that the healthcare system should be kept at its present size and in its present configuration, given utilization rates and trends. Convulsions have shaken many other economic sectors in this country that were once considered untouchable: horse-drawn transportation, railroads, lumber, printing and publishing, and defense, to name a few. It is healthcare's turn.

And it does not seem either logical or moral to keep useless, low-quality services open when they are not being used, or when they are not being used enough for them to be safe and efficient. Healthcare is too expensive to serve simply as the site of make-work employment.

Who Should Be Protected?

So should we then, in the words of Marc Antony in his elegy for Julius Caesar in Shakespeare's great play, just "cry havoc and let slip the dogs of war"?

We can't. There's a difference between eliminating "feath-erbedding" jobs on the railroads and closing a town's only hospital, between reducing a junk-bond dealer's income to only a few million dollars and condemning a low-wage healthcare worker to unemployment, poverty, and even homelessness. Allowing huge numbers of "losers" in healthcare can mean unacceptably high losses to too many other people.

I think there are several types of potential losers we need to worry about, for their sakes and our own:

Low-echelon healthcare workers. Healthcare is a bit unusual in that someone can do a specialized job—say, being a home health aide—and still be paid quite little. Especially in hospitals, the workforce in central sterile supply, security, dietary services, housekeeping, and the like have more training than low-paid workers in other sectors, but are extremely vulnerable to being laid off and having trouble finding new jobs.

This workforce is disproportionately female and minority, and includes a higher-than-average percentage of single mothers. Compassion would dictate that we not just throw them to the wolves of unemployment.

Underemployed or unemployed physicians. Depending on whose figures one uses, in a completely reconfigured system we could have between 100,000 and 250,000 excess physicians. Although many nonphysicians are less than sympathetic about this, and although medical schools deserve recrimination for having produced too many of the wrong kinds of physicians for a quarter-century or more, physician underemployment and unemployment represent a major public policy challenge.

These professionals will need retraining, redirection, and redeployment, none of which will come easy for a profession whose members are traditionally independent, entrepreneurial, and change-resistant. For those who have earned enough and paid off the mortgage, early retirement or part-time work might be a solution, but for those who are still carrying large debt and who have children to educate, something must be done.

If we ignore the problem, remember the words of John E. Wennberg, MD, who has been studying this issue for some time: "In a market with an increasing supply of resources and particularly of physicians themselves, one should not underestimate the ability of physicians to come up with new ideas." The question is whether those new ideas would benefit patients—or endanger them.

Necessary services. Some hospitals, clinics, nursing homes, physicians, and other providers are indeed essential. So are services such as trauma care, burn care, child abuse treatment, care of those who cannot care for themselves, and public health activities such as vaccination of children. The problem is that these services add to the cost structure of whatever provider offers them, thus making the provider less competitive in a cost-driven market. In rural areas, some healthcare services are equally necessary, even if they operate at less than peak efficiency under urban definitions.

It is utterly necessary that we define which services are truly essential, and that we protect them, paying whatever extra price is required. In some cases, this might involve subsidizing what market-oriented economists would call "fat." But even economists, I suspect, would not be comfortable about being run over by a truck in a community where the hospital with the only trauma center had closed because it was considered too costly.

Vulnerable patients. Although one hears less and less about it as the reform debate becomes completely monetarized, the fact is that at the heart of healthcare is a very intimate, delicate, and emotional transaction between a sick or injured person and the individual who is taking care of him or her. Reform allegedly seeks to strengthen that relationship by recasting its context in a saner, more responsible, and more resource-sensitive mold.

Reforms that instead cast certain patients onto the trash heap because they are not profitable or powerful or attractive are not reforms. They are acts of bigotry and profiteering, and they have no place in healthcare.

Four Lessons

How, then, might we protect these potential losers? By borrowing four lessons from our own history and from other sectors that have faced similar dislocation:

1. Allocate resources for redirection. It is not as if there is no need for skilled labor in this country, in and out of healthcare. The retraining and redeployment of workers—professional or not—who have been displaced is entirely possible and has been accomplished repeatedly. Certainly the federal government has been throwing money at the retraining of redundant defense workers, just as it has funded the retooling of many defense industries into energetic and productive civilian firms. We should do no less for those who have worked in healing.

2. Do community health planning. Sorry to bring up a dirty word, but somebody has to figure out what sort of healthcare system we want to have. So far it has been a hit-and-miss matter, relying far more on factors such as wealth, aggressiveness, and pitiless competition than on community wants and needs.

The concept of planning fell on hard times in the Seventies, when it was perverted into a sleight-of-hand (and largely unsuccessful) exercise in cost containment. It needs to be revived, in the form of community leaders—business, the public, payers, government, and providers—sitting down and asking, "What do this community and region need? What do we have? What needs to be protected? What should be closed or converted?"

Yes, there will be terrible fights in the course of making those decisions, and politics and influence will take their toll. It won't be a tea party. But it would be far better than the survival-of-the-fittest approach we are taking now, which promises to produce results that would make Darwin pale.

3. Consider the consequences. A growing consciousness on the fragility of our earth and the need to protect it led to the development of a new evaluation tool during the Seventies and Eighties: the environmental impact statement. This describes what the effects—good and bad—of a planned project are likely to be, and how they will interact with the environment. It seems to me that we should similarly try to assess the impact of the restructuring of healthcare financing and delivery, with an eye toward preventing destructive and unwanted results before they occur, as well as for spotting trends that should be encouraged and warning signs that should be heeded.

4. Monitor the results. If there is one thing we have learned in this century, it is that all policy is imperfect. No one—save the elite in their ivory towers—really thinks that the implementation of fancy untried economic theory, the reversal of payment incentives, and the revamping of the delivery system will go like clockwork. We are going to make a lot of wrong guesses, go down a lot of blind alleys, and foul a lot of things up.

It is therefore our responsibility as a society and as a healthcare sector to monitor, evaluate, and disclose the results of what we do as we re-create ourselves. This is not something we are good at, as a people. We tend to have a short attention span, and once something has been done, we try to forget about it—until the roof caves in because of mistakes and problems we ignored.

The stakes in healthcare reform are too high for us to pursue this sort of here-today, gone-tomorrow philosophy. We cannot hide the evidence of failure when we encounter it simply because we don't want to let go of cherished ideas that we wanted to work. We have to learn from our successes and our errors as we go through these profound changes, and we can only do that if we track their effects.

If we are willing to learn from where we have gone right and wrong, then the casualties of reform can be minimized. If we are too busy living for the moment to consider the kind of future we are creating, then we will all be the ultimate losers.

A Gift of Trust

November 1994

Trusteeship, if you think about it, is a pretty strange job. I mean, people who may or may not have management or governance experience are asked to take responsibility for a large, often multi-million-dollar entity, for little or no pay. And it's part-time work!

If you posted that job description in most places, people might doubt your sanity. Yet thousands of people accept and pursue this difficult and often underappreciated work, year after year, and have done so since the beginning of organized healthcare in this country.

It's Not What It Used to Be

Needless to say, trusteeship has changed over the years. We all knew of instances in which a board position was purchased for, say $1 million for the building fund (and some of that still goes on). Membership on certain boards was more dependent on which country club (if any) one belonged to than whether one was actually bringing anything to the position. Board membership was sometimes almost hereditary; commonly, when a male board member died, his wife was invited to replace him, as though it were her birthright. In fact, at one time, these women represented a large proportion of female board members who were not members of religious orders. Too often, however, they were seen and not heard, and were relegated to the meaningless safety of the lawn and garden committee.

Things are different today. Some changes were inevitable, such as the healthcare organization providing liability insurance for board members, and the now-common practice of paying trustees something for their time. (That pay, of course, can be outrageously high, which to some of us seems incompatible with the idea of voluntarism, but that's another column.)

Moreover, as hospitals, physicians, group practices, hospice programs, nursing homes, and other providers join together both vertically and horizontally, the trustee's role has been altered. Where once the board was composed of local folks charged with the governance of a local institution or organization, today the board may have responsibility for providers hundreds or thousands of miles away. That original community board might be three levels down from the top, with a charge that is little more than advisory.

Two other changes in trusteeship are equally profound. The first has to do with the fact that, traditionally, most healthcare boards were dominated by white upper-class men (although a few boards, interestingly, are mandated to be all women). That is not to say they have not done a good job: many have, and some have not. But the demographics of our communities have changed, and the healthcare workforce has come to include many more women (more than 80 percent) and minorities. As a result, there has been increasing pressure for more heterogeneous boards. This has proven to be easier said than done.

Second, the concept of community is being redefined in our changing healthcare world. Once it was the local area; now it might be a community of like interest, such as women, patients who are HIV-positive, people of color, or those who favor a single-payer healthcare financing mechanism. As a result, what constitutes a community board, and who/what that board is supposed to represent, has become a fluid concept that is ever more difficult to define. Not surprisingly, board members find themselves at odds with each other more often, and boards find themselves at odds with their communities more than ever.

On top of all this, attempts by healthcare organizations to find capable trustees, and signals from capable people who wish to serve on boards, often seem to miss each other. And for those entities whose boards are elected (mostly public and district hospitals, although it is also true of some HMOs and other organizations), this already tricky process is bedeviled further by politics.

Hey, it's a tough job, but the pay's lousy. . . .

Diminished Trust

Much can be said about all this, but a couple of thoughts seem most relevant. The first is that the word *trustee* has as its first syllable the word *trust*, and much of what is making trusteeship so problematic these days has to do with the public's diminished faith in providers and insurers. If you don't trust the organization, you won't trust its board.

This year's (and last year's and next year's) debate over healthcare reform has, of course, exacerbated problems of trust, because it has been an exceptionally ugly fight. Vicious broadsides have been launched against insurers, physicians, hospitals, HMOs, politicians—you name it. Providers are greedy, insurers are interested only in profits. HMOs deny access to care, and so forth and so on. Such allegations are not likely to increase public trust in providers and payers.

I don't think this is going to turn around anytime soon. This is a consumerist age, and a distrustful one. This year marks the twentieth anniversary of the resolution of the Watergate scandal, which was a key factor in reducing the American public's trust in many of its institutions. Use of tough business and industrial terms, overaggressive marketing and competition for patients, egregious profiteering, and the reaping of massive personal fortunes within healthcare, along with the familiar issues of patient dumping and overbuilding of huge, expensive structures (often with little thought as to the effect on the neighborhood) have not helped matters.

So at the very time that many providers are trying to restrain unproductive competition and work together for community betterment, many communities are less trustful of them than they have ever been. The result is that their efforts to communicate with each other badly miss the mark.

A Huge Gap

My other observation is that there is often a huge gap between good-faith efforts and effective results, and nothing illustrates that so clearly as the gulf between provider organizations' efforts to diversity their boards, and the outcome of those efforts.

For it is not just the healthcare world that has changed. Today, 60 percent of American women hold jobs outside their homes. The postponement of childbearing means that many women in their forties and even fifties have young children. There are more single mothers than ever before. This is a far different female talent pool, in terms of potential trustees, than the stereotypic (and unfair) traditional image of "Mrs. Gotbucks" and her bridge partners.

Recruiting working-class folks and people of color to board membership can be even more problematic. There are all the issues that any candidate faces in terms of available time, childcare problems, family demands, and the like. There is also the fact that society is more racially and socially divided than it was a generation ago, largely because of housing and education patterns.

There are probably more successful people of color today than has even been the case. But the ability of healthcare boards to find and recruit them, and retain them once they have accepted board positions, is limited. Often they just travel in different circles than traditional healthcare trustees.

In addition, when a woman or a person of color, especially a younger one, does gain visibility in the community, he or she is often overwhelmed by offers to serve on boards. I have several African-American women and Latina friends who have been asked to join so many boards that they could probably attend a meeting every night for a month and not repeat! The answer, it seems, is in casting the net farther, rather than in everyone trying to compete for the same two or three candidates.

That also applies to seeking younger trustees, which is difficult. In addition to having lower levels of experience, many young people, no matter what their color or gender or social level, see healthcare trusteeship as a hobby for old fuddie-duddies. Their voluntarism is more commonly directed toward environmental and personal causes.

Of course, not everyone likes the idea of women and people of color and young folks and community activists serving on healthcare boards. It does tend to upset the status quo. There are cultural conflicts to overcome, power struggles to sweat through, and sensitivities—often extreme sensitivities—to deal with.

I am reminded of the time I attended a conference, years ago, at which there was one woman speaker. She was terrible. The head of the organization that sponsored the conference told a colleague of mine, after this woman's dreadful performance, "You see? Women speakers aren't any good."

Too often, board members feel the same about folks of different sexes or cultures or ages or political persuasions who come onto boards and upset the apple cart. So they seek to remain safely within the white-upper-class-male (conservative) mode, because they believe that is where the greatest expertise lies—while those watching them conclude that they are racist, sexist, and elitist.

All this is going to take a long time to sort out, and few boards will make it through that time without getting bruised. However, it seems to me that there are a few things a healthcare organization owes to its trustees, and a few things a trustee owes to the organization on whose board he or she sits. Perhaps serious consideration of these principles can make the experience a little less bloody.

What Does the Organization Owe the Trustee?

1. Honest information about why he or she has been asked to sit on the board. Just as, too often, we train young physicians in settings that have nothing to do with the realities of medical practice, so we often are not direct with potential trustees about what we want from them.

We praise their intelligence and talent, but we really want their money. Or we say, "You were the best person for the job," but we think, "Oh, boy! An African-American woman professor!"

We also tend to underestimate how much will be required of the potential board member, which leads too many new trustees to drop out after a while because they do not have the time. The more realistic the presentation, the more likely a gifted trustee will give the time and stick around.

The demands of trusteeship can also be less overwhelming if we ensure that childcare (or parent care) is available; that meetings are held, as much as possible, at times that do not conflict with professional or family responsibilities; that modern technology such as teleconferencing is used to minimize the number and length of face-to-face meetings; that committees and subcommittees are used effectively; that travel is minimized; and that staff support is first rate.

2. Realistic empowerment. The relationship among trustees, administration, and medical staff has always been something of a three-way tug-of-war. However, the time has passed when the board could function as a rubber stamp, blithely approving anything the administration and physicians wanted. This kind of ineffectuality proved disastrous in terms of physician credentialing, levels of organizational debt, and community relations; no organization can afford it today. Besides, a strong board that knows its powers and uses them wisely is the best friend administrators and physicians can have.

3. Assistance in dealing with various communities. In a world where more than one community is served by a provider—where, in fact, people in many states may be members or patients—boards at all levels of the organization need to tread a fine line among competing interests. They need to be aware, therefore, of issues being put forth by community representatives, and they need counsel as to the strength of feeling behind the issue, the importance of the issue to the organization, and the probable consequences of this or that decision.

It is no favor to the board not to mention that ACT UP representatives are sitting in at the enrollment offices, claiming that the HMO refuses HIV-positive patients. After all, it was some hospitals' and physicians' cavalier treatment of the uninsured sick that led to federal and state anti-dumping legislation, and it is some HMOs' overly tight concept of accessibility that is damaging managed care's image. The board needs to know where problems exist, so it can address them.

4. Respect, gratitude, and friendship. Trusteeship can be rewarding, prestigious, and productive, but it is not always fun. Those who serve on boards have a right to be treated with respect. Yet we still hear of CEOs who view the board as an enemy or an obstacle to be gotten around. Board members deserve gratitude as well, which can be expressed in a variety of meaningful ways, not just with wall plaques. Perhaps most important, trustees should be treated as friends of the organization; if they are not, what are they doing on the board?

What Does the Trustee Owe the Organization?

1. Reasonable commitment of time and talent. Board membership is not a bauble, yet too many people wear it like a piece of jewelry, using it as a resume item or a means of making professional contacts. The organization has the right to expect trustees to devote a reasonable amount of time and talent to their duties. This may or may not mean completely faithful attendance at meetings, but it does mean making a significant contribution. If you cannot make that contribution, you should resign.

Last year, I was removed from a board I should have left voluntarily. I have finally learned not to accept board service in the first place, because my schedule usually prevents me from properly discharging the responsibilities involved.

2. Honesty of agenda. One of the most common and often most destructive, events in trusteeship occurs when a person with a narrow agenda runs for or seeks selection for a board seat. Once on the board, the person desires only to pursue his or her private cause. This can be anything from a social agenda (women's or gay causes, for example) to a personal one (a desire to get a particular administrator fired, which I have seen succeed).

On the one hand, the complaint may be legitimate, in which case the board should hear the person out and try to remedy the situation; but this one-note approach cannot be allowed to go on, meeting after meeting, for years and years, to the detriment of the board's other work.

Certainly, any trustee is entitled to personal areas of interest; that is why many people seek to join boards. Indeed, physician and nurse board members are often expected to represent their colleagues. However, there is also a duty to the organization and to the larger community. One must strike a balance, and trustees who refuse to do so are best invited to leave.

When that person represents a popular cause, or is a woman or a member of a minority or otherwise protected group, there can be hell to pay. But just as there are disruptive physicians, there are disruptive board members, and there must be safeguards against them. Their ill behavior, however, does not mean that their causes and interests are automatically invalid: it is usually the messenger, and not the message, who is the problem.

3. Acceptance of change. Boards are often conservative, and that is probably how it should be; as I often say, I would not be terribly happy being a patient of a faddist hospital or radically experimental physician. However, under too many board tables, one can see the marks where heels have been dug in repeatedly, often long after change should have been accepted.

These are volatile times in healthcare, and unresponsive organizations, or those whose boards still long for the good old days, are unlikely to flourish—or, in some cases, even to survive. Conservatism and resistance to change are two different things, and board members need to know the difference.

4. Respect, gratitude, and friendship. The hours are often long, the work difficult, and the rewards problematic. Nonetheless, even as one is wading through the alligators, it is important to remember that trusteeship is a gift that goes both ways. It is still an honor to serve on a board, even in these troubled times, and that honor should be returned with respect for the organization, gratitude for the opportunity to serve, and good feelings (to the degree possible) for those with whom one works.

In coming years, some boards will have to shut down their organizations; others will merge into larger entities when they would have preferred independence: still others will face radically different missions and scopes of work. Yet even in facing and implementing such difficult decisions, trustees should keep in mind that voluntary service to a charitable enterprise has long been considered one of the highest forms of work in this country. One hopes that board members are aware of that, and are grateful, just as we should be grateful for their guidance.

I've Got a Secret

January 1995

A candidate for mayor in Chicago is confronted by reporters asking about his earlier hospitalization for depression; the information was leaked by someone at the institution where he was treated.

A candidate for vice president of the United States is forced to withdraw his candidacy after news comes out that he had suffered from depression and had undergone electroconvulsive shock therapy.

A candidate in a congressional race in New York City wins her primary, after which records of her psychiatric treatment the previous year are leaked to the press.

Arthur Ashe—athlete, historian, statesman, teacher—is forced to reveal at a press conference that he has tranfusion-induced AIDS after someone (Ashe believed it was a healthcare worker) leaked the news to a national newspaper, which then informed Ashe that it was going to publish the story with or without his permission.

And we have hardly begun to construct the healthcare information superhighway. All this, and thousands of similar transgressions, happened in a time of minimal computerization and paper medical records.

What on earth will happen when the integrated electronic medical record becomes the norm? When a patient's medical records can be called up on any of 200 computer screens within a large, comprehensive healthcare system?

Although his proposal was not passed by Congress, President Clinton presaged the future when he waved a "health security card" and promised that all Americans would have one—complete with the data strip on the back that would tell providers (and insurers, and alliances, and employers, and others) all they wanted to know about the owner's health status and interactions with the health-care system.

Healthcare often has a good time with technology. Whether it's imaging systems or laparoscopic surgery or genetic medicine, physicians and nurses and hospitals and systems like incorporating new machines and procedures into their work. And anything that is thought to make providers' and patients' lives easier is enthusiastically accepted.

This tells me that the electronic medical record is a sure thing, sooner or later. Indeed, a 1993 survey conducted by Hewlett-Packard and the Healthcare Information and Management Systems Society revealed that 52 percent of healthcare professionals polled thought computerized medical records would be a *fait accompli* within five years. That's now three years.

Would that be such a disaster? Well, I raised the issue of patient information confidentiality with representatives of some major HMOs last year—organizations that are well on the way to having such systems—and to my surprise, one physician stood up and said that she utterly opposed the movement to computerize medical records. She said that the data simply could not be protected sufficiently, and that the risk to patients was too great. (I think it was no coincidence that she works in an area where AIDS is a full-blown epidemic, and I know she is not alone in her beliefs.)

However, on the other side are arrayed a powerful set of advocates of electronic patient records and large computerized patient databases (as well as computerized databases containing information about providers). They include many health insurers, who wish to know what risk any given policyholder or applicant might represent; indeed, one of the more unfortunate public relations campaigns launched in recent years came from a group of commercial insurers who promised, "The less your risk, the lower your rates." Translation: "The greater your risk, the higher your rates—if we decide to sell you coverage at all." No wonder that the one aspect of reform that virtually all states and (allegedly) most members of Congress agree on is reforming a health insurance system that discards you if it finds out you are sick.

The insurance question is complicated, to be sure. My point here is simply that many insurers are very interested in data about patients, and not all insurers confine themselves to legally acquired information. Furthermore, there are persistent rumors about a database shared by insurers that is said to contain health status information about millions of people; all that can be confirmed is that there exists a database with information about people who have withheld information or lied on their insurance applications.

Researchers I have talked to strongly suspect that it goes way beyond that. Of course, if inaccurate information about an applicant or policyholder went into such a database, it would be extremely difficult to correct the data if those in control of the database denied that it existed.

Who Wants to Know?

Stomping on commercial insurers is easy. But I do believe that federal insurance reforms will be passed relatively soon, especially because many states have already enacted such legislation, to one degree or another.

But it isn't just the commercial insurers. Others, too, are looking for information. Outcomes researchers, seeking in all good faith to find out which treatments and procedures work and which don't, need information on thousands of patients. Of course, the information base does not need to identify individuals, but in the course of checking accuracy and doing other things to enhance the integrity of the work, researchers may need to peep into people's personal files. Even if the names are blacked out, coded, or removed, privacy can be at risk.

Peer reviewers checking on the necessity and quality of patient care need to see records. Utilization reviewers need to see records. It would be a blessing to trauma teams and emergency department staff if they could get instant information about the comatose patient lying before them, who may or may not be allergic to penicillin.

Employers who are paying for care often want to see records, and, of course, employers who sponsor employee assistance programs are themselves in possession of potentially damaging information. Even if the information is not about impaired employees, it can provoke totally inappropriate responses. There was the case, a couple of years ago, of the employer who learned an employee who carries the gene for cystic fibrosis was pregnant. The employee was informed that she would no longer have insurance unless she had an abortion.

And in the notorious McGann case, about which I have written before (in the September/October 1993 issue), the U.S. Supreme Court upheld the right of a self-insured employer to retroactively deny benefits to employees who contract AIDS.

And the age of genetic medicine is coming quickly. Already, we can test for a number of genetically linked conditions that might predestine a fetus for a short, sick, and expensive life. As the project to map the human genome—to identify and determine the effect of every gene in our bodies—progresses, we will identify genes that can lead to a predisposition to cancer, alcoholism, muscular disorders, diabetes, and neurological diseases.

Soon to be nailed firmly to the wall, with tests to follow: genes associated with hereditary nonpolyposis colon cancer, at least one form of breast cancer, one form of ovarian cancer, and Alzheimer's disease. Already in use: tests for cystic fibrosis, Huntington's disease, and several other rare conditions.

In other words, a lot of folks want to know what we have and when we got it and how we got it and what we did about it, and not all of them are acting in our best interests.

It is, therefore, not surprising that the public has its doubts. A September 1994 survey by CNN and *Time* magazine found that 65 percent of the public thought genetic engineering was not a good idea (26 percent thought it was). If the technology was used to cure disease, however, 79 percent approved; 16 percent did not. Use of genetic technologies to simply improve a person's appearance was opposed by 70 percent of respondents; 25 percent approved. But 90 percent opposed use of such information by insurers.

How Do We Do It?

The question at the core of all this is: How can patient information be protected so that it is used only to benefit people, and not to penalize or harm them because they are sick?

This is going to be one of the key debates of the Nineties, and possibly *the* debate of the first decade of the new millennium; it was even a part (although, sadly, a very small one) of the debate over healthcare reform in 1994. It is a topic we will all undoubtedly return to, time and time again.

Nonetheless, I would offer a few thoughts as a sort of early warning system:

1. Make protection of the privacy of patients and co-workers part of the culture of every healthcare organization, no matter its size or scope. Healthcare has a long way to go before it can say it is doing a good job even with the information it has now. One CEO told me that when he joined his organization, it was commonplace to wheel medical records around in shopping carts. If the courier wanted to stop for coffee or to use a restroom, he or she would just leave the cart out in the hallway, vulnerable to anyone's inspection.

The CEO started kidnapping the carts and keeping them in his office until word got out that a cart was missing. Sometimes he had half a dozen of them. To retrieve the errant cart, the courier would have to visit the CEO's office. Medical records security got tighter in a hurry.

Another hospital leader hands out cards stating that patient privacy is the highest priority of the institution—a written promise to patients. That pledge is taken by every new employee.

Incorporating protection of privacy into the culture means training new employees, and continuing education for incumbent employees. It means formal sanctions for violation of confidentiality rules, and informal sanctions in the form of consistent, meaningful disapproval of idle gossip or malicious conveying of information. In other words, if someone in the cafeteria starts talking about which patient had an abortion or tested positive for HIV, everyone around him or her should tell the offender to shut up.

2. Enact legislation and regulations that protect private information about people, no matter how it is stored and collected: on paper, in computers, or over fiberoptic phone lines. The federal Privacy Act of 1974 requires federal government providers to gain patient permission before releasing personal medical information about them, but not all states do the same; indeed, only 27 states mandate that providers allow patients to see their own medical records.

There are some federal protections for patients in substance abuse programs that receive federal funds, but again, other providers are often not included. And, as consumer advocates have pointed out for years, patients are often asked to sign long, vague informed-consent statements that allow just about anyone access to their records—except, in many cases, themselves.

The very first kind of legislation and regulation we need is insurance reform that makes it irrelevant whether an applicant or policyholder or employee is sick or well, or carries genetic time bombs. It is disgraceful that our health insurance system has become so perverted that those who need coverage the most are often least able to obtain it. Even if we had universal coverage, discrimination against the sick (who are, after all, more expensive, which is a disadvantage in a capitated payment system) would be a danger. In the absence of universal coverage, with insurance risk-rating the order of the day, being sick can be a death sentence.

We need both state and federal statutes that can be implemented, have meaningful penalties, and are enforced, even if the offenders are powerful insurers or political operatives.

3. Start talking to each other about what information is really necessary, how it should be collected so that privacy is preserved, and how it can be protected. This means everyone involved: the research, provider, and data collection communities. Part of the emergence of health services research has been a sort of obsessive national search for healthcare data, regardless of whether those data are going to do anyone any good, whether they have any research importance, and whether anyone can make heads or tails out of them. We need to figure out what is really useful, who needs to know it— and how to keep it private from others.

4. Affirm the right of people to see their medical records, plain and simple. Concerns about malpractice attorneys or others conducting "fishing expeditions" cannot serve as a barrier to people finding out about their own treatment and experiences.

Besides, anyone who is contemplating a lawsuit can get hold of any records that exist; it is only the hapless patient who might be curious, or who wishes to correct inaccuracies, who gets frozen out.

5. Create technologies to protect information that has been collected and stored electronically. It is undoubtedly possible to do so. Despite the powerful interests that would wish it otherwise, such protections must be developed, disseminated, and used religiously.

6. Close the loopholes to the degree possible. There will always be loopholes. There will always be hackers who think it's fun to break into other people's databases and fool with them; there will always be those who are willing to provide information for a fee; there will always be those who will delight in using confidential information to humiliate, threaten, and blackmail others.

Our job is to keep those people at bay to the greatest extent possible, through a systemwide commitment to protect every piece of information about a sick patient, a positive test result, or an impaired physician or nurse as though it concerned us or our family members.

The issues are complex and troubling, as in cases of child abuse, transmissible disease, or potentially harmful, impaired providers, but we can work through them. The two overriding principles are simple enough: First, the welfare of the patient must come first, hell or high water; second, unless I understand and agree otherwise, my healthcare secrets are none of your business.

A Sense of Loss

March 1995

It is the classic physician's or nurse's dilemma: The patient cannot be cured or stabilized. She (or he) is going to die. Yet the patient demands that treatment—futile though it is—be continued. Or the family demands that useless treatment be initiated or continued, with or without the patient's agreement. The latter most commonly occurs when the patient is no longer competent to express his or her wishes, and has not left any written directive. In some instances, family members may disagree among themselves as to what should be done.

The other scenario is discussed less often: The patient can be saved by proper treatment; a cure is probable. The treatment may be unpleasant, but it works. Yet the patient refuses it, sometimes without giving a reason for doing so.

In both cases, the problem is the same: The physician or nurse or hospital does not believe the patient's or family's stance is well advised. Even in a healthcare environment that respects patients' wishes—and we like to think that most providers work in such an environment—this situation is frustrating and sometimes infuriating. And often, no amount of discussion or counseling among the parties concerned can resolve their differences.

This dilemma is brought up more than any other by physicians and nurses with whom I discuss ethics problems. In my experience, the tendency of providers (which is understandable) is to grouse about the stupidity or stubbornness of the patients and families. How can they demand wildly inappropriate treatment? How can they refuse treatment that could save their lives and restore their health?

The first, and obvious, comment is that if the patient is competent, he or she has a perfect right to refuse anything he or she does not wish to experience; I think that is accepted by most physicians and nurses. The situation is much messier when the requests or refusals involve the care of a child or a person who is not deemed competent. Nonetheless, competent patients have the last word, even if it literally is their last.

That principle, however, does little to smooth the emotional topography of the nether land of inappropriate demands and incomprehensible refusals. So providers get frustrated and angry, and patients and families get more obstinate, and sometimes the whole thing ends up in court.

One question does not get asked enough: Why do people make irrational demands? The usual arguments are that families feel guilty and patients fear death, that lay people believe that even a 1 percent chance of survival is reason to act (as in the case of the conjoined Lakeberg twins), that Americans are not willing to take "no" for an answer. In other words, they just don't understand.

It's more complicated than that. The reasons are different in each case, of course, and the forces that underlie demands for overtreatment differ from those that underlie refusals of appropriate treatment. But we can identify some common motivations, which might help us understand and ameliorate the complex pressures and emotions that are at work.

Demands for Overtreatment

There are at least five underlying causes of such demands.

Fear of abandonment. Eminent healthcare philosopher Daniel Callahan has theorized that one reason patients make irrational demands for healthcare that cannot benefit them is their fear of abandonment. He is absolutely right. In a healthcare system whose values are derived from a curative model that embraces the acute and shuns the chronic, a model that rewards the cure while disdaining palliation, it is little wonder that a patient who is dying believes that if he or she gives in to that dying, the healthcare system will abandon him or her. Patients thus fight to stay within the acute, curative model, even if it will do them no good whatsoever. Few of us want to die alone.

The great British health policy analyst Rudolf Klein has pointed out that whereas Britain is something of an "original sin society" that sees death as a natural part of life, the United States is a "'perfectibility of man society' in which illness and debility are seen as challenges to action." If you are dying, you fail the test; you are of no further interest.

No wonder that Callahan has suggested that the highest priority in healthcare should be concern and caring for those who are not going to get well. Should we ever widely adopt such a culture in healthcare, patients' fear of abandonment would diminish greatly.

Suspicion about providers' motives. In the old paternalistic days, if a physician said, "There's nothing more we can do," that was it; you started planning the funeral. Today, patients might respond, "Does the HMO give you a year-end bonus if you come in under budget?" One of the sadder consequences of our monetarization of healthcare is that the public is much more aware of providers' economic motives and conflicts of interest. People thus become wary when told that further treatment is inadvisable.

Certainly many of those who advocate for patients with AIDS and breast cancer believe that the healthcare system has dragged its feet in terms of finding more effective and less disfiguring treatment. More than a few people have expressed cynicism about the convenient availability of donor organs to celebrities and politicians;

indeed, one rather paranoid novel suggested that there are dark goings-on in organ transplant programs (and it has been demonstrated that all has not been entirely kosher in some of those programs). At a time when public trust of providers seems to be heading south, it is not surprising that patients and families do not always accept providers' claims that further treatment is futile.

Belief in the power of technology. Professor William Sullivan, among others, has stated that Americans like to produce technical solutions to social and emotional problems. I tend to agree; I think that's why the powerful moral and social aspects of the healthcare reform debate disappeared in a hail of econometric bullets. It is therefore logical that Americans would seek to create technological answers to flesh-and-blood problems, and that is just what we have done in healthcare. Our industry is wedded to its technologies, and we have conveyed that passion to the society at large. As a result, most people think that there must be a technological salvation—a new drug, radical surgery, an experimental approach—even when none exists.

Intolerance of the imperfect. This society exults in the Body Perfect—young, blond, thin, exquisite skin, bright eyes, firm muscles. That standard does not mesh well with the lesions of Kaposi's sarcoma, the weight gain associated with immunosuppressives, the loss of a limb. Those with serious physical or mental conditions are less socially acceptable than the rest of us. Those who are in constant pain—and there are millions of people who are—become a pain for the rest of us. They are the healthcare homeless, always among us, objects of pity whom we wish would go away. They and their families therefore demand that the healthcare system return them to membership in the club of "normal" people.

Inability to confront the mysterious. No matter how and when it happens, death is the most mysterious of experiences. Although a

few people claim to have been there briefly, no one has ever come
back after, say, a year or so to tell us all about dying and being dead.
It is an unfathomable process. It is, for one thing, a solitary journey;
it reflects the line of the song that goes, "You've got to go to sleep
alone/Even if you're lying with someone you really love/You've got
to go to sleep alone." The body stays with the living; the soul
departs. And it is a permanent separation, at least in this life.

No wonder that we embrace the ideas of afterlife, of ghosts, of
visitations from the dead. The person who is dying has slipped the
traces of normal human existence; he or she is utterly beyond our
control. No wonder that families, facing the total loss of both their
power over and their relationships with the dying person, try to
postpone that moment of truth.

Refusal of Useful Treatment

In a landmark article in the *New England Journal of Medicine* on
August 23, 1979, David Jackson, MD, and Stuart Youngner, MD,
issued a set of warnings about patient refusal to accept life-sustain-
ing treatment. To this day, their concerns are highly relevant:

- The patient is ambivalent about surviving.

- The patient is suffering from clinical depression (which
  goes widely undiagnosed, especially among the elderly).

- The patient is actually seeking help for another problem.

- The patient is afraid of the treatment or technology
  that would be used.

- The patient's family disagrees with the patient's wishes
  for continued treatment.

- The provider assumes that the patient wishes no further treatment when that is not the case.

THE RIGHT THING

This is a very useful litany of reasons why patients and families go against rationality and, often, the best interests of the sick person and/or the family. I would like to examine more closely a few of the fears underlying some of these reasons:

Fear of being a burden. Most of us are not cheered by the prospect of being dependent on family members or others in our last days, or of being chronically dependent on anyone, or of being a drain on the family finances. This stems not only from a terror of loss of independence, but also from a humane fear of unduly burdening those one cares about.

As a result, patients may well opt out of further treatment because of concern for their families and friends and the economic, logistical, social, or emotional burden the patient might place upon them. This happens to be a legitimate concern, but in most cases, a more benign alternative than premature death is available. We can learn a great deal about such alternatives from the formal and informal volunteer programs that have done so much for AIDS patients during the last decade.

Fear of pain. This is certainly one of the key issues that lead patients to reject further treatment, and that is tragic. As one hospice physician told me, one of the down-sides to the anti-drug campaigns of the past 15 years is that many physicians are hesitant to prescribe sufficient quantities of painkillers—even if the patient is within days of death. I am aware of brutal examples; a good friend of mine, who was dying of cancer, ended up in an emergency room in agony one night because his physician didn't want to put him on methadone "too soon." The problem was that morphine had ceased to be effective.

A survey by the Eastern Cooperative Oncology Group, published in the *Annals of Internal Medicine* on July 15, 1993, found that 86 percent of the physicians surveyed believed that most patients with pain received insufficient medication. A troubling 49 percent of respondents reported that their own pain-control practices were subpar; 18 percent said they were poor or very poor.

Patient reluctance to report pain was cited by 62 percent of physician respondents; the same percentage reported that patients were reluctant to take opiate drugs. But 61 percent of the physician respondents said they were reluctant to prescribe opiates, even when appropriate. This hardly reflects state-of-the-art management of pain. But, as the authors note, "Pain control has historically been a low-priority issue in cancer care."

And providers wonder where Jack Kevorkian came from.

Fear of technology. As has been observed often, healthcare technology is a two-edged sword (or a two-edged laser knife, perhaps). On the one hand, patients and families often demand it inappropriately. On the other hand, patients and families are often cowed, if not downright terrified, by the huge machines, the toxins and poisons, the lasers and neutrons, and much of the rest of the armamentarium. They are not unaware of side effects like nausea, hair loss, scarring, and burns. They also usually receive insufficient counseling about the technologies, how they are used, why and how they work, and why they are being recommended in this particular case.

As a result, they spurn the machines and drugs and operations, often for very good reason: They're scared stiff of them, even more so than they are of death.

An electronics firm's television advertising campaign includes the slogan: "Hey, we make technology people want." I don't think they make radiation oncology equipment.

An Underlying Loss

All these reasons, and dozens more, contribute to patients' and families' making decisions about treatment that most physicians and nurses find inadvisable, if not lunatic. But there is one thread that runs through all of them: a fear of disempowerment.

340 THE RIGHT THING

In the end, the presence of Death lurking in the corner reduces the power of everyone else in the room. Death disempowers those who are sworn to heal and makes them feel less "in charge." Death disempowers family members who no longer have any control over their relationships (resolved or not) with the dying person. And, ironically, death—or its prospect— can empower a patient who has been rendered powerless by disease or injury; I am told that there is an enormous sense of liberation in knowing you are headed out the door of life.

Thus it is the gaining or losing of power that often determines what a physician, nurse, patient, or family member will decide. Until we recognize that, we will continue to question each other's choices without really understanding them.

* * * * * * *

Easing the Final Task

Having had more than my share of experience with serious illness and death among my friends and family members, I offer a few thoughts to those who are going through the dying of those close to them:

- *People who are dying are still people. Often what hurts them most is that those around them do not know how to deal with them. The fact is that they are the same folks they always were; they're just sick.*

- *People who did not like being patronized or fluttered over when they were well are not likely to enjoy it any more now.*

- *People who are confined to bed get bored, especially if illness or medication affects their eyesight. They may appreciate the gift of a cassette player with book or music tapes. You might ask if they would like you to read to them. They might just appreciate the company, even if you're just sitting there, reading a book.*

- *Some people who are dying welcome help in planning rituals such as wakes and funerals; in deciding what should happen to their possessions (often they prefer to give them away while they are still living, so they can enjoy people's reactions); and in creating scrapbooks, videos, and other remembrances for family members.*

- *People who are dying do not need to worry about the four food groups; they are not building a strong and healthy body for the future. So forget about being dietetically correct and find out what sick folks would like to eat. Of the gifts I have given, one of the more appreciated was a case of fresh Hawaiian papayas for someone who could not keep other food down because of medication.*

Sigmund Freud once wrote, "Toward the person who has died we adopt a special attitude, something like admiration for someone who has accomplished a very difficult task." It is up to those of us who love the dying to keep that task from being any harder than it has to be.

. . . .

This column was dedicated to the memory of Frank Sabatino, former editor of Hospitals & Health Networks, *who died on January 7, 1995, at the age of 46.*

If You Really Mean It

May 1995

Although we tend to think of healthcare as a staid, stable, and largely conservative (socially and politically) sector, the fact is that we are just as given to fads as anyone else. In only the past few years, we have been through corporate restructuring, competition, collaboration, reform, and integrated delivery system formation. We are in the second cycle in 15 years of aggressive for-profit hospital activity, as well as the second cycle in 20 years of Medicaid managed care. There was even a brief flurry of renewed calls for closure of public hospitals, which was as short-lived as the 1994 push for universal coverage, to which Congress turned a deaf ear.

Healthcare providers seem to have a weakness for me-too-ism, even if the fad is fleeting, and even if the model being touted is not appropriate. After all, "managed competition" among HMOs is hardly appropriate to Alaska, where there are no HMOs , and small community hospitals lost a lot of money during the Seventies and Eighties on corporate restructuring that had little or no effect on their activities. It just seemed to be the thing to do.

On the other hand, all these trends had promise, and some yielded great results—mostly when providers recognized the limits of the models, applied the lessons appropriately, and were sincerely committed to change.

Healthy Communities: Just Another Fad?

We are now seeing a wave of interest in "healthy communities"—the notion that a healthcare organization has a responsibility to protect and enhance the health of all those it seeks to serve, whether that population is defined as people living in a given geographic area, people with a particular diagnosis, people with specific needs, people who belong to a given health plan, or people who hold particular values or beliefs. All these are definitions of community, as I outlined in a previous column (*Healthcare Forum Journal*, May/June 1993).

This idea is not new, indeed, under the name "population-based medicine," it has been a hallmark of managed care for many years. Elucidated by healthcare sages from the late Rufus Rorem to Merwyn Greenlick of Kaiser Permanente, the concept is that it is the health plan's (or provider's) duty to always consider the entire population for which responsibility is undertaken. In the case of some HMOs, unfortunately, that came to mean that the HMO was interested only in its own members, but in many other cases, there was a strong community commitment.

The re-emergence of interest in this concept lately has many sources. One is that several key health status indicators for Americans are discouraging. Although white infant mortality continues to decrease somewhat, the figure remains much higher for children of color. Longevity has stalled, although the quality of life for people over 65 continues to increase. More children are dying from violent causes than ever. More Americans have AIDS and are HIV-positive. Any physician, nurse, hospital leader, group practice manager, or health plan executive can see that our rather narrow, medicalized model of healthcare is not even beginning to reach the kinds of problems that are out there.

Another reason for the push toward community health, I suspect, is that with the increase in HMO membership (now more than 50 million Americans) and capitated payment, the financial incentives of health status are reversed. When piecework ruled healthcare, providers made more money from sicker patients. With flat-fee payment, the provision of health services is a source of cost, not profit. When early HMOs were being accused of everything from communism to neglecting patients, they often used this same argument: If we ignore patients' health until they are very sick and need hugely expensive care, we lose money. It seems the healthcare field is finally starting to understand this line of reasoning.

I must add that early intervention and health promotion are not the hallmarks of all managed care plans or capitated payment arrangements. Some plans simply shove all the risk onto providers and stroll away, counting their cash. Others make access so difficult that even basic health services go by the board. And some entrepreneurs make their money by setting up plans, signing up members, and then selling the plans before the big bills start coming due a few years down the line.

Nonetheless, managed care and capitation provide a powerful reason for keeping one's patients and members healthy.

A third reason that the healthy communities concept is becoming popular is the explosive growth in larger healthcare organizations. Although most of them call themselves *integrated*, some are and some aren't. Those that are encompass a variety of services, from outpatient primary care to inpatient services to long-term care to home care to hospice. When the entire continuum of care is the responsibility of a single organization, it does not take long to realize that the earlier the intervention in the course of illness, the less the stress on the patient and the system. And when inpatient hospital care is just one of many services provided, there is no reason to value it more than others.

It would be naive to ignore a fourth reason: The increasing pressure on hospitals and systems (and in some cases, health plans) to justify their tax-exempt status and demonstrate the benefits that their communities derive from their activities. From California to Massachusetts, Utah to Pennsylvania, state and local governments are getting a lot tougher about what constitutes community service on the part of healthcare providers. And as Congress seeks to reduce federal funding for human services across the board, and slip the unpaid bills to states, counties, and cities, pressure on providers and plans will only increase. Although embracing community health may thus be a cynical move on the part of some providers to avoid paying taxes, there is no reason that it should not produce positive results.

Finally, there is a growing interest on the part of many Americans in improved personal health. Many forces are feeding it. One was a string of outspoken surgeons general—C. Everett Koop, Antonia Novello, and Joycelyn Elders—who made smoking and reproductive health very public issues (and all of whom were punished to one degree or another for their stands). Another is that the first baby boomer turns 50 in 1996, and there is a sense of desperation as bodies sag and bellies enlarge. Also, some practices are no longer seen as acceptable; certainly smoking has been made not only unfashionable, but also difficult, with social, financial, and legal sanctions in place in most states (this is such a strong trend that I suspect attempts by tobacco-belt congressmen to reverse it will not succeed).

So there are sound reasons for the healthcare field to become more heavily involved in population-based, community-oriented healthcare. Many of them already are: the list of recent winners of the McGaw Prize for community service reads like a Who's Who of socially responsible healthcare organizations. In other cases, however, the commitment may not be there; instead, it may be a case of follow-the-leader, or else opportunistic exhortations by consultants and others who see a gold mine in this movement.

How to Practice What You Preach

I have spent a great deal of time in recent years with providers who do practice what they preach, and who really are committed to community health. I have gleaned much from those visits and discussions, and have based a series of principles on what I have learned. These are not rules or standards; every community is different, and every community health effort is different. But they might prove helpful in evaluating a program to ensure that it really is meaningful in the long run.

1. If we undertake to care for a given community, we care for all who are in it. Their race, gender, age, diagnosis, social station, lifestyle, or culture should not matter. Many of us mumble about universal access and coverage, but we should understand that universal means exactly that: No one is excluded. That can often mean tailoring programs for people who are different, whether we approve of them or not—and asking them to participate in program design and implementation.

2. Financial barriers are not the only obstacles. The healthcare system has erected many nonfinancial barriers that exist even if potential patients are insured. When heart disease in women is under-diagnosed and little researched, when people of color have less access to cardiac and kidney care, when people diagnosed with diseases like HIV or chronic mental illness have nowhere to go in the system, that is not an insurance problem: that is a community problem.

3. Waiting for those who are in need to come to you is lazy and ineffective. Providers often condemn patients who do not seek preventive and early-intervention care as stupid and "non-compliant." However, if people who should be using your services do not do so, there are many possible reasons. They may have no transportation, they may have no childcare, they may be afraid of abusive spouses, they may be too proud to seek healthcare handouts. Community-oriented care means reaching out, not just sitting around waiting for whomever walks in the door.

4. Addressing nonmedical issues is part of the solution. Poverty, violence, hunger, prejudice, malnutrition, homelessness, lack of self-esteem, and hopelessness are all sources of poor health, just as surely as lack of immunization is. I once asked the director of an urban public hospital why the institution had such a large dental service. He responded, "People who are malnourished and eat out of garbage cans have bad teeth." And people who have no reason to believe that they will live to see the age of 21 because of the violence around them are unlikely to become honor students and keep their bodies pristinely healthy. Some of these problems are very hard to combat. It's easier to medicalize the situation and just wait for them to be carted into the emergency room.

But I learned a powerful lesson from George Adams, president of Lutheran Medical Center in Brooklyn (a McGaw Prize winner), years ago. I asked him why the hospital offered courses in English as a second language. He answered that he had many immigrant patients who did not speak English: "Although many of them have good job skills, they can't get good jobs if they can't speak English. If they can't get jobs, they can't get health insurance. If they can't get health insurance, they can't pay me. It's just self-interest on my part." It was a lot more than that. George Adams was a pioneer in community healthcare and is passionately committed to it. His reasoning simply strengthens the argument that healthcare is more than a technical, clinical affair.

5. Dignity and charity are not mutually exclusive. It is part of human nature, and part of American social tradition, to be charitable in some manner at some point in our lives. It may mean nothing more than plunking a dollar into a Salvation Army kettle, or it may mean spending a year working with Mother Teresa. However, too often this giving has a patronizing edge to it, the lingering aura of noblesse oblige—of superior beings deigning to share a crumb with their lessers. It reminds me of the retort issued by the late writer James Baldwin when a society lady in New York City assured him that she gave her African-American maid all her cast-off clothing. "Very well," replied Baldwin, "and does she give you hers?"

Honoring the dignity of those one serves should be part of all service, even though sometimes it can be mighty tough. In community health efforts, respecting the dignity of others can mean the difference between success and failure. Too much current health promotion is highly judgmental, and often reflects an attitude of "I'm better than you are because I don't smoke," or "I'm too smart to have an unwanted pregnancy." Just because people are struggling with poor health practices does not mean that they are a lower form of life. Those of us who have been blessed with good education and financial stability and a desire (and capacity) for self-improvement should keep in mind that we are very lucky; most of the world does not have such advantages.

6. No one individual, nor one community, can do everything. It is difficult to believe that one is doing much good when the tasks seem overwhelming. But it is important to remember the Dean Witter principle: "We measure our success one investor at a time." Sometimes, community health efforts can only be measured one member of the community at a time—and that may be years after the fact. But as I try to stress to state legislators and health officials, every life we protect, every little program we initiate, every piece of insurance reform, every small act, is a victory. No one effort, no one program, is going to save everyone. We can only do as much as we can, and join hands with those who are doing the same, and one day we will find we have accomplished a very great deal.

7. Long-term accountability means everything. Early victories are pretty easy. It's not rocket science to raise the immunization rate a few points. With minimum effort, more prenatal care can be made available. Getting Yuppies to do a few more sit-ups is not an overwhelming challenge. The temptation is to hit the easy, cheap problems and populations.

But out there are also homeless people with disabilities, addicts who have had bad experiences with detoxification programs and are suspicious of them, people whose culture is so alien you can't figure it out, people who are involved in illegal activity—people you don't approve of and who probably don't think much of you, either.

The further down the road you go in search of community health enhancement, the harder it gets. The problems get tougher, and it becomes more difficult to keep existing programs vibrant and meaningful. It is then that we have to think very deeply about our accountability.

Unless we are willing to submit ourselves to the scrutiny of the communities we seek to serve, and unless we are willing to demonstrate that we actually made a difference, our claim of commitment to community care is simply a gimmick. It means that we are afraid of asking for the judgment of the community. It means that when the going got tough, we went shopping.

Obviously, few of us want to be accountable; it's scary. But I cannot think of any other way to find out if what we are doing is doing anyone any good. That is why I am so impressed with John O'Brien, chief executive officer of Cambridge (Massachusetts) Memorial Hospital—another McGaw Prize winner. He and his staff identified several groups in Cambridge (including young men of color) whose health status was at risk and who were not being reached by the hospital's existing programs. O'Brien then made his future raises— his very income—dependent on whether these groups could be helped, with real, quantifiable improvements.

Similarly, Group Health Cooperative of Puget Sound includes improvement in member health status in its annual report. This is, if you will, a social corollary to the "report card" movement that calls for comparative outcome data reporting by providers and health plans.

8. Be patient. Some improvements in community health can come quickly, but building the social, scientific, and spiritual infrastructure necessary to keep improving and to prevent backsliding takes a long, long time. What is needed is a program and a commitment that can survive shifts in the political and fiscal winds, that can accommodate changes in fashion and mores, that is strong but still can be recreated all the time. Whenever you think that you are far enough ahead to give it a rest, remember that every day a child is born who will take everything you have done for granted and ask, "What have you done for me lately?"

It can be a long, hard road, and often an unrewarding one. You will never see some of the fruits of your labors. (I often think Louis Pasteur would be astounded to see his name plastered on milk cartons boasting that their contents have been pasteurized: he probably never thought he'd end up as a common verb.)

But those fruits will grow, and foster more improvement, and upon that foundation will someday be raised healthier, happier, safer children. What we do today will come back to us, in time. As musician Richard Thompson wrote in his elegy for a dead friend, "If you really mean it/It all comes 'round again." And if we really mean it, the story of our communities will be found, in part, in how hard we tried to protect each other.

Just Another Day at the Office

July 1995

The CEO was tired. It had been a long teleconference with the CEOs of other units in the system, and despite the ergonomically correct individual tele-headsets on which the conference was broadcast, her head hurt. Probably eyestrain. She chuckled; maybe she should sue for workers' compensation! After all, injuries related to computers and electronic communications were now far and away the most common workers' comp claims.

It was a long cry from the Nineties, when back injuries were the most prevalent claim, and chiropractic the most used workers' comp service. Today, it was proton/laser ophthalmology and electromagnetic-orthopedics—two board-certified specialties that had not even existed when she first went into health administration.

She switched on her voice mail. It began reciting her messages in a low, soothing voice—a voice that still reminded her of HAL, the talking computer in Stanley Kubrick's film, *2001*. She had mentioned that to her administrative resident, Chakira, who just looked at her blankly. The CEO had then remembered that the resident was born almost 30 years after the film was released; it had no more meaning for Chakira than the films of Tom Mix had had for the CEO when she was in her twenties.

Nonetheless, the CEO had nicknamed her voice mail apparatus "HAL."

Blond, Blue-Eyed Males

HAL presented her messages in that velvety voice: "Message One: The Genetics Subcommittee of our hospital's Joint Medical Staff-Nursing Staff-Board-Administration Patient Protection Committee has issued its recommendations concerning the System's involvement with cosmetic genetic manipulation of sperm- and egg-bank donor stocks. Would you like a summary?"

The CEO nodded. She was grateful that HAL could respond so quickly to nonverbal signals; that last upgrade to instant visual recognition had really helped.

"Summary as follows: The System, in accordance with federal, state, and local laws ['all we needed was local home-rule authorities getting involved in health policy,' the CEO muttered], recognizes that genetic science can improve the prospective health status of fetuses through altering of eggs and sperm, as well as postponing, moderating, or even stopping the course of certain diseases in children and adults. The System has been supportive of, and has participated in, these advances—although it continues to be apprehensive about societal, employer, and health-plan discrimination against those persons known to be at higher risk of genetic disease.

"However, the System cannot support the use of scarce societal and healthcare resources to guarantee that the use of anonymous egg- and sperm-bank donations will result in 70 percent blond, male, blue-eyed fetuses. The System therefore should decline to participate in such programs."

Besides, the CEO thought, *the child population of the suburbs around here looks like we're in Scandinavia, not the United States. And the dearth of female children is destroying girls' sports programs in the schools.*

But then, because all school sports programs had to be open to children of both sexes, only the voluntary all-girls programs in the private schools were being affected. The public schools had had to abandon sports programs when, in 2005, Congress folded all education funds into block grants for the states. Her state had spent the funds on suburban schools and building prisons.

She dictated a brief memo to HAL:

"To: System Patient Protection Committee, Mayo-Ecumenical-
          MegaHealth System
From: CEO, Memorial Hospital Unit, Western Region
Subject: Cosmetic Genetic Manipulation of Sperm- and Egg-
          Bank Stocks

"Herewith the recommendation of our Unit's designated committee on the subject issue. We urge the System to adopt the position
we have taken. Best wishes for the Generic Holiday." (One could
no longer offer specific religious greetings over interstate business
communication lines.)

She told HAL to send it to the System committee's office, where
it would be printed out and distributed electronically to all the units
in the System in a matter of seconds. *Sure doesn't leave much time for
corrections or second thoughts, does it?* she mused.

Ethics in the Service of Economics

The soothing voice spoke again: "Message Two: The Executive
Health Administration Program at the University called. Will you
be giving the annual administrative ethics lecture this year?"

She told HAL she'd get back to it/him on that. She wasn't sure
it was worth it. Ever since all health administration and health policy programs had been folded into the economics departments of
participating universities in 2010 (at the insistence of then-Com-
merce Secretary Alain Enthoven, under whose authority all healthcare activities and funding had been placed after the abolition of
the Department of Health and Human Services), her enthusiasm
for teaching the social aspects of healthcare had diminished.

It wasn't that the Commerce Department was not trying hard
to have a balanced curriculum for health administration students;
indeed, the department had issued guidelines for ethics and social

content. It was just that, at the local level, many of the economics professors had not had much ethics training themselves, and therefore were poorly equipped to teach in this area.

The shift of health policy from a broad social, economic, and philosophical focus to a strictly economic one during the Nineties more or less dictated that administration students be prepared for a totally budget-driven environment. Still, she wished ethics and mission were core curriculum subjects, instead of electives. The lecture she gave each year was sometimes the only ethics content that the health administration students received—and there were few things as dreary as giving a required lecture, during which a certain percentage of the students were sure to be doodling, daydreaming, or simply sleeping.

Many of the students, of course, worked to fill in the gaps in their education. The elective ethics courses were always popular, and many master's and doctoral theses were devoted to the most serious of ethics and mission topics. Chakira, for example, had written her thesis on social barriers to health services and health careers for Americans of diverse racial heritage.

The expansion of federal civil rights legislation during the presidency of Joseph P. Kennedy II had theoretically protected virtually every identifiable ethnic group, as well as women and homosexuals, although compliance was spotty. But no one had thought to include Americans of varied heritage, who fell into no Census Bureau category. That had, of course, led to the embarrassing incident in 2002 when Eldrick (Tiger) Woods—the brilliant golfer of African-American, Asian, and Caucasian heritage—won the Masters Tournament but was not allowed to play later that year at a golf course near Chicago.

In healthcare, as reports and monographs continued to show, the situation was just as bad: Although access and coverage were allegedly color-blind, members of minority groups (who, in some areas, were no longer minorities, but dominated the population) still had less access to a wide range of health services than did majority groups.

Nonetheless, we have to keep trying, she thought. "Sure, HAL, tell the University I'll give the lecture." The best hope for improving health administration education, after all, was involving more practicing professionals in faculties that were distressingly short of real-world experience.

Life Enders

"Message Three: Six more members of the medical staff and eight more nurses are refusing to participate in patient-requested suicide or patient- or provider-instigated euthanasia. The Oncology and HIV services are very thin on physicians and nurses willing to participate. Can you meet with the board on this soon?"

She told HAL that she would, of course, and asked it/him to go over her schedule and make an appointment for later that week. HAL immediately scheduled the teleconference and listed the date and time on her electronic wristwatch/calendar/phone.

The law said that patients could request assistance in ending their own lives at any time, although dissenting caregivers could refuse to participate. But the paperwork for filing a refusal was cumbersome, and some physicians and nurses felt that by refusing, they were abandoning their patients at a critical time. The standards for euthanasia—physicians and nurses terminating patients' lives directly—were tougher, but a lot of it was still going on. And there had been a nasty case when the medical staff of the HealthTrap HMO were encouraged by the corporate owners to end the lives of elderly cancer patients, almost all of them women.

When the inevitable lawsuit followed, the HMO argued that euthanasia was far more cost-effective than hospice care for terminal cancer patients. Several Medicaid programs—which were largely under state control now—immediately sought federal waivers to offer cancer patients the option of euthanasia over hospice care. The National Hospice Organization sued to prevent the waivers from being granted. The whole mess was now at the U.S.

Supreme Court. She wondered what Associate Justice Lance Ito, now the swing vote on the Court, would decide.

But all that was for the high and mighty. She was just an executive of a 150-bed teaching hospital—quite large for an inpatient facility in the year 2020—and her nurses and physicians were increasingly resistant to ending patients' lives on demand, especially for reasons of cost containment.

She sighed. She would probably have to contract with Life Enders, Inc., the proprietary physicians' group who would terminate any patient for a percentage of the capitation. Many other provider organizations had already contracted with them; it was so much easier than fighting the medical and nursing staffs.

Still, it made her uneasy. *We are all going to die, and most of us will be sick or injured when we do*, she thought. *Debility shouldn't be a capital offense.* She was glad her husband had died in a hospice program years earlier.

Alzheimer's: No Treatment Required

"Message Four: George says that the Resource Allocation Committee has been unable to come to a decision about continuing the Alzheimer's Day Program. Looks like you'll have to decide, or else kick it to the Board."

We should have seen it coming, she thought. With all public and most private health expenditures capped and capitated, the payers had placed all the risk onto providers, forcing them to make the hard decisions. Yeah, sure, there was allegedly a basic benefits package for which all patients were eligible, but it was *so* vague: What did "basic inpatient services" or "demonstrably effective primary care" mean?

It would have been so much easier if the outcomes movement of the Nineties had not been stalled as a result of lawsuits by alternative therapy providers and mental health professionals, who claimed they could not come up with outcomes data, as well as by lawsuits from patients who felt they had been denied potentially effective therapies. Of course, by the turn of the century, there was such a massive oversupply of specialists and nonphysician providers that many of them were eking out a living as professional witnesses, and you could always find someone who would testify that *any* therapy was potentially helpful.

As it was, even those health services known to be effective—such as immunization against measles, the common cold, and some strains of HIV—were not always available, because there was little or no oversight of compliance by health plans and providers with the basic benefits package. And if a plan didn't happen to have a high immunization rate, but was a dollar or two cheaper per month, well. . . ?

So the children, the poor, the chronically ill, and the elderly suffered. Especially the demented elderly—most of them poor, alone, and female. Now the commercial insurers had sued over the expense of treating Alzheimer's, and the disease had been dropped from the very short list of specific conditions for which treatment was required. Payers were eliminating coverage for the disease. The argument was that Alzheimer's patients had lived their lives, more or less, and money was needed for the young.

But we aren't taking care of the young, either, she fumed. *When the state of Oregon started reducing the number of Medicaid services available to welfare families,* she thought, *I wonder if they thought it would end up like this.* Not surprisingly, Oregon was also one of the leading states in physician-assisted suicide and euthanasia. If the hospital was going to continue the Alzheimer's Day Program, she would first have to convince the board that it was a good idea, and then they would have to snip here and there from other programs to find the money. This was something around which they could raise philanthropic funds as well, probably. She wished she knew more about how to ration care in a responsible manner.

She knew one thing: She would not abandon the elderly patients who flocked to this unit. It was one of the few that still treated them with respect. Indeed, one of the proudest possessions of the unit was the beautiful handmade quilt that its elderly patients had made and given to the hospital. The unit had loaned it to the Alzheimer's Association for its quilt project, and it had traveled the country. She was glad it was back. She felt a need to go look at it, to remember what handwork and folk craft and individual creativity were about.

A Brief Tour

She told HAL she was going to walk around, and it/he activated the beeper on her wristwatch/calendar/phone. It, too, spoke when she was paged, but in a flat electronic voice, not HAL's lovely tones.

After looking at the quilt for a while, she went to Oncology to visit patients she had met earlier. Anna Wilson had chosen euthanasia, and was gone. Even with all her uneasiness about the process, the CEO was glad that Anna was no longer suffering.

Robert Chang was still there, surrounded by friends and family. The CEO was so pleased that she had been able to fully integrate hospice into the capitation rate. She stopped in to say hello, and was rewarded by a big smile from Robert and his family members. *At least we have really good pain-killers now, and every physician and nurse knows how to use them. Not like the old days, when palliation was a rare skill.*

The Nursery was busy, as always. All the baby boys in their bassinets, with adoring parents hovering nearby. She stopped to look at one child: a beautiful little girl with honey-colored skin, almond eyes, and dark hair. *I hope we have some of this stuff figured out by the time you are my age,* she whispered silently.

She was glad there was still room for people to be different. She remembered a field of daffodils she had seen in the Skagit Valley of Washington state, on a bulb farm. Daffodils stretched as far as the eye could see, until they met the fields of tulips at their edges. In the middle of the daffodils stood one red tulip—defiant, different, daring anyone to make it be a daffodil. A lovely intruder.

On her way back to the office, she stopped by the Emergency Department. Controlled chaos, as usual. Two young men had attacked each other with laser shotguns; their burns were being treated, but one had been blinded.

The nurses were tending to a confused homeless man. They knew him well, and even kept a medical record on him in the integrated computer network. They could do at least that much.

There had been a minor AirTrain monorail accident. The emergency staff, professional to the hilt, were evaluating and triaging the victims. They would all survive, but Laser Surgery would be busy tonight.

At the far end, an old man was dead—coronary, probably. His insurance company undoubtedly was already figuring out how much should be deducted from the payment to his widow, based on his apparent violations of the Correct Eating Act of 2008. A physician was explaining to her what had happened and was offering the unit's help. A nurse cradled the woman's head, stroking her hair as she wept. The staff were respectful of the moment, understanding that even in these techno-times, death was the most private of mysteries. The entire scene looked like a religious tableau, reminding the CEO of a Renaissance painting.

She turned to go back to her office. Her wristwatch beeped. It was HAL: "I figured you would want to know. The Cubs are losing to the Mets, 17-2."

Some things never change.

* * * * * *

I would like to thank David Hoskinson, vice president for managed care, Catholic Healthcare West, for one of the ideas in this essay. He knows which one.

Something in Common

September 1995

Americans, it has often been pointed out, are the most individualistic of creatures. Indeed, the very word "individualism" was coined by the French social analyst Alexis de Tocqueville in his exhaustive 19th-century study of American society and character. Many other students of sociology, psychology, and the mentality of nations have observed the same about us: We don't like to stand in lines; we don't like to be told what to do; our individual rights are very important to us.

And, of course, we are very uneasy about our relationship with government, because government necessarily infringes on those personal rights. Although Americans' suspicions about their elected and appointed officials are being used at the moment to feed ideological and political agendas, the issue goes deeper than partisan politics. It has to do with the fact that this nation was founded by anti-government radicals, and their shadow still hangs over us today.

Remember that 30 years ago, it was left-wing radicals, not right-wing white supremacists and militias, who considered the federal government to be their sworn enemy. A few of them even engaged in terrorism, although nothing so awful as the Oklahoma City bombing.

So our individualistic streak runs both broad and deep. And right now, that streak is on full display as a national debate (or what should be a national debate, anyway) rages over how healthcare for the elderly, the disabled, and some of the poor should be funded. The same debate has erupted about welfare and food stamps and a number of other social programs that seem to fly in the face of American individualism, in that they use tax money to subsidize services for people who, by and large, are not paying all that much in taxes. In other words, taxpayers, so the argument goes, are not getting back, in services or whatever, what they are putting in.

The same issue is front and center on the state level as well. In my adopted state of Illinois, for example, there are always two civil wars going on. One is a fight for control of resources between the cities and the suburbs; the other is the same fight between rural and urban areas. These battles sometimes are fought along party lines, and sometimes cross those lines. They are never resolved to anyone's satisfaction.

The Many and the Few

What is really going on here is something that is key to any restructuring of healthcare delivery and financing: the degree of cross-subsidization we are willing to tolerate.

You see, virtually all tax-funded activities and virtually all insurance are based on a simple principle: Money is drawn from the many and targeted to the few. It doesn't matter if the arena is agricultural policy, defense policy, or health policy; the principle is the same.

Although most of the population of the United States is now considered urban, taxes from all of us go to subsidize farmers, including those who grow tobacco, which most of us do not use. (Until two or three years ago, we were subsidizing the production of mohair, because it was once used for military uniforms and nobody ever got around to repealing the subsidy.) Money from all of us supports the defense industries and the armed forces, although opinion is certainly divided about whether we all benefit from everything they do.

And money from all of us goes to support the 70 million people—elderly, disabled, those with end-stage renal disease, certain low-income families with children, many nursing home residents, and others—whose healthcare is funded in part or totally by the Medicare and Medicaid programs. Furthermore, because employment-based health insurance premiums are not taxed, those who do not have insurance or who must buy individual insurance (most of which is not tax-exempt) pay taxes that are needed to make up for the taxes that are not assessed on group policies. This is one of my favorite ironies: The uninsured working poor are actually subsidizing the health coverage of the insured, working well-to-do.

But then the insured population, in one way or another, is subsidizing the care of the uninsured poor, when they can get it, either through artificially high insurance premiums that reflect cost shifting by providers or through tax subsidies that keep open the last line of defense, our public hospitals. And, of course, individual policyholders subsidize the cheaper policies issued to groups.

On the delivery side, profitable services subsidize unprofitable services in hospitals and clinics (a transplant program, for example, might help support a busy trauma center), and, in at least some multi-provider systems, profitable hospitals and clinics may subsidize other members of the system that are not so fortunate.

In other words, healthcare financing is a game of taking from Peter to pay Paul, or sometimes taking from Paul to pay Peter. It is an intricate web of cross-subsidization.

But Is It Fair?

Is this a good way to pay for health services? There are arguments on both sides. Certainly, there are ethical and moral problems with "hidden subsidies"—cost shifting, overcharging, cooking the books, and other games providers have come up with to cover the costs of caring for the uninsured and, in some cases, Medicaid and Medicare patients.

But as long as the nation refuses to set up a system whereby people who cannot afford to pay for insurance or for care can get both at a price they can afford (and most of them cannot afford anything to speak of), providers can argue that they have been stuck with the bill for an incomplete insurance system, and they thus have every right to scrape up the money to cover the costs by imposing involuntary subsidies on payers.

Still, it does seem kind of sneaky to jack up a heart surgery bill to keep the emergency department functioning.

Insurance carriers, on the other hand—with the exception of many HMOs—do not believe in cross-subsidization when it comes to pricing premiums for applicants who are not members of large employee groups. That is, if it seems likely that you may cost more in terms of health services utilization, you will be asked to pay a higher premium—if they are willing to sell you a policy at all. Or else the policy may exclude the organ system or condition that is making you sick.

This is known as risk rating, and it is very consonant with American individualism. In fact, in a notorious series of newspaper ads a few years ago, the commercial insurance lobby informed readers that "the lower your risk, the lower your costs." Translation: The higher your risk, the higher your costs.

This is certainly a logical application of the principle of individualism, and as more and more data appear on genetic predisposition to disease, insurers will be able to risk-rate ever more accurately.

So even in the seemingly mundane world of health insurance, the specter of individualism rears its ubiquitous head.

And in our current political and moral climate, the battle cry is seductive: Free the individual to make his or her own decisions! Return power to the states! Stop the government from interfering in our lives (with the exception of certain circumstances in which people with political axes to grind want the government to outlaw this or allow that). The Senate passes a bill allowing states to post whatever speed limit they want, and to stop federal sanctions against states that do not have mandatory motorcycle helmet laws. Between the two, many thousands of people will die or become seriously disabled (and we will all cross-subsidize that, too).

States want to trim their Medicaid rolls, with special attention being paid to getting rid of "welfare bums," most of whom are young mothers and children whose healthcare costs are minimal—but who are being subsidized by the rest of us. Most Medicaid spending is on nursing home residents, the low-income elderly, the disabled, and the blind, but don't tell that to those who are sick of subsidizing welfare families.

This is a familiar turn of the wheel of fate: We range from "rugged individualism" to a "welfare state" in terms of what the national philosophy *du jour* is, and we demand that government honor whatever that philosophy is this week.

Three Slight Caveats

I would offer three slight caveats in the face of this.

First, we should keep in mind that the American public does not view health insurance as an exercise in risk rating. Opinion polls show that Americans see health insurance as an exercise in risk spreading—that is, everyone throws a certain amount of money in the pot, and those who are unfortunate enough to need it draw out what they need. This was the original basis of insurance, and it became especially important for healthcare because one never knows when an adverse health event might strike, what it might be, or what will be needed to alleviate it.

So whether it is public or private coverage, this notion of only putting in what you will pull out, or of basing premiums on health status or genetic traits or "deservingness" or whatever, inevitably leads down the darkest of one-way streets: Insurance will fail to operate. No one but the healthiest, with the best genes, will be able to acquire coverage, and the stressed public sector and emergency rooms, whose cost-shifting capacity is increasingly limited, will crack under the strain.

The end-point of this is medical savings accounts, whereby the healthy can bail out of health insurance altogether, leaving the sick with premiums they cannot afford.

Community rating—charging everyone the same premium, regardless of other factors—is, in the end, not just an easy way to price insurance. It is the only way that insurance can survive as a private means of paying for healthcare.

My second caveat is that trying to destroy publicly funded social programs because the government went into big-time debt during the Eighties will not work. If Medicaid and Medicare are cut to pieces or egregiously underfunded, what will replace them?

Can destitute African-American women in their eighties suddenly start paying premiums to Prudential? Will a cabdriver's family suddenly be able to come up with $4,000 for a premium? Can this country ask the healthcare system to pick up the unpaid bills for tens of millions of newly uninsured people?

Are we prepared, in our individualism, to let the aged and sick poor die in the street on the grand scale, as opposed to the minor scale on which they do so today?

Of course not. And if we are unwilling to do that, then it seems to me that the best—if not the most politically feasible—approach is to accept that cross-subsidization of some Americans by other Americans is necessary in order for third-party payment and tax policy to work.

So maybe we should just all heave a sigh and accept government attempts to redistribute some of our money—even if it means that some of us may draw out more than we paid, which is true of many people over 85, because they were nearly at retirement age when the Medicare trust fund was established.

That does not mean that wild profiteering by payers or providers, or overuse of the programs by thoughtless beneficiaries, or fraud by anyone should be tolerated. It just means that if we try to declare that it's every man and woman for himself or herself in healthcare, we might as well fold our tents and go home, because we will collapse our system.

My third caveat is that there is an ethical as well as a fiscal and logistical reason to accept cross-subsidies in healthcare. That reason, as has been argued by Howard Hiatt, MD, and George Annas, JD, is that healthcare is not 253 million different, individual situations; healthcare is a commons. The very nature of hospitals, physicians' practices, clinics, nursing homes, and other places where people care for other people is that of a sharing place, of something we all have in common.

Where did people go when the federal building in Oklahoma City was shattered? Why do rural communities scrape and claw to keep little hospitals open? Why do we all fear the closing of an emergency department?

Because we know that healthcare, in the end, is something that we all share, even if we don't all use it. Indeed, except for preventive care, most of us would prefer to have as little to do with being patients as possible. But we need to know it is there. We need to know that "loser" burn and trauma services, 24-hour coverage, the seasoned wisdom of an experienced specialist physician, and the quick wits of paramedics are there when we need them.

And like the parks that bear the name "commons," healthcare thus necessarily must be supported equally by those who need it and use it and those who are fortunate enough not to. It must have the resources to do what it needs to do, regardless of party politics, insurance theory, economic ups and downs, and all the slings and arrows of a participatory democracy.

And that means that we must stop blaming the beneficiaries for overusing Medicaid and Medicare; that we must look very hard at how healthcare money is distributed and spent, so that we can reduce unacceptable levels of fraud and profiteering. And we must put one principle above all the ideological harangues of the day: The reason we consider our healthcare system to be among the best in the world is that we all share it; we all have a sense of ownership of it. And thus, we all must protect it from those who see it as just one more individualized commodity.

Good healthcare respects the individual; good healthcare encourages individual responsibility; good healthcare is provided on a personalized, individual basis. But good healthcare, in the end, is only good when it is also something that is shared, across time and place, by all people.

Never Again

November 1995

As it draws to a close, we should look back on 1995 as a year of extraordinary history. It was the year the United States reopened its embassy in Vietnam after 20 years of pain and controversy. It was the year that saw the fiftieth anniversary of the dropping of atomic bombs on Hiroshima and Nagasaki (and may those be the only two times such weapons are used in human history!). Of course, 1995 was also the year of the fiftieth anniversary of the end of World War II. It marked the one hundred thirtieth anniversary of end of the Civil War and the death of Abraham Lincoln, and the seventy-fifth anniversary of American women winning the right to vote. And on September 6, Cal Ripken, Jr. played his 2,131st game as a Baltimore Oriole.

Healthcare and social policy had their own historic moments this year. On July 30, we noted Medicare's and Medicaid's thirtieth birthdays (although almost all the celebrating was over Medicare, with little attention paid to the equally important "other" program). On July 14, a brutal heat wave hit the city of Chicago after four mild summers; by the time the temperatures had abated, 733 people were dead of heat-related causes. On August 9, guitarist Jerry Garcia of the Grateful Dead died in a drug treatment center of an apparent heart attack. And on August 13, baseball legend Mickey Mantle died of widely metastasized cancer nine weeks after receiving a liver transplant.

I suspect this year will be remembered for a very long time, in and out of healthcare.

I also suspect that, as happens far too often, the lessons of history in which this year was saturated will go largely unlearned. Americans, as historian Arthur Schlesinger has pointed out, are not exactly infatuated with their own history, and the politicization of history teaching by forces on both the right and the left hasn't helped. History seems to be losing its credibility with the public.

Even if one has a sense of history, once one gets into healthcare, it takes no time at all, apparently, to learn what a medical society lobbyist observed earlier this year: "It does not pay to have a long memory in this business." We in healthcare have a huge capacity for ignoring the past, with the result that we repeat our mistakes, time and time again. We go through ebbs and flows of concern for the poor and vulnerable, sometimes seeking policy solutions for their plight, sometimes condemning them for their own weakness and seeking to abandon them.

We engage in cycles of overbuilding hospitals, and then wake up one day and say, "Gee, we have a lot of excess capacity. I wonder how that happened?" We have an unbelievably ambivalent relationship with managed care and capitation, in some years seeing them as the perfect solution to healthcare's woes, and in other years viewing them as some kind of communist plot.

But we seem curiously unable to see the patterns that these cycles form, or to break those patterns when we need to. Instead, we often act like mice on a treadmill, doomed to repetition.

The Lessons of '95

I do not think that the lessons of 1995 can be dismissed by healthcare, however, and so, as the new year looms, I would like to outline some of them—along with some suggestions for New Year's resolutions for all of us.

The Death of Jerry Garcia

I went to college in Berkeley during *those* years (1964-68), and I remember the emergence of the Grateful Dead as part of the entire folk-rock movement, which was part musical innovation, part political expression, and part (a large part) drug use. It was anti-war marches and flower power all mixed up together, and we romanticized it.

And many people continue to romanticize it—in fact to yearn for the days when you could get away with anything and still feel that you were on the side of the angels. Rose-colored memories feed our need to still rebel, and it is even easier when we can do so vicariously through celebrity rebels.

The problem is that few people can get away with everything and stay alive and healthy; time and your body catch up with you. Garcia was the latest in a long string of vibrant musical artists whom we have lost to self-destructive ways of living: Billie Holiday, Charlie "Bird" Parker, Hank Williams, Elvis Presley, Janis Joplin, Jimi Hendrix, Jim Morrison, Kurt Cobain, and many more. The wonder is that Jerry Garcia lived so long.

Yet our response is always the same: We shrug off their deaths with a fatalistic belief that nothing could be done to deter them, or else we condemn them as negative role models who have a corrosive effect on our youth. In some cases, we continue to romanticize them: One troubling example was Dan Ackroyd at John Belushi's funeral, declaiming that "great talent allows great excess." No, it doesn't, Dan; that's why John is dead.

It is not easy to succeed with health education for adolescents and young adults; often, part of their finding their own identities is engaging in behaviors that we more seasoned individuals know are dumb or dangerous. But I don't think we can give up. We have seen a massive shift in attitudes among the middle-class young when it comes to smoking and drunk driving, and, in many cases, illegal drug use. We need to learn why and how we have succeeded, and extend those lessons to other behaviors and to other youth subcultures.

Let us resolve that if we are going to talk the talk of prevention, we should also walk the walk, and that means confronting social and cultural factors that encourage slow suicide.

An Epidemic of Heat

The wave of death that overtook elderly, chronically ill, and homeless Chicagoans in July and August was not the first. In 1980, equally dreadful weather led to the deaths of some 1,500 elderly people across the country. Many lost their lives in St. Louis. That city initiated a program for preventing such a calamity from happening again, and healthcare providers there became involved in prevention efforts. Other cities, especially Chicago, did not get the hint.

Centuries ago, we recognized that cold was a killer; but heat was generally a friend. There were ponds and lakes and rivers to cool off in, and Native Americans knew how to construct lodgings that warded off extreme temperatures. When air conditioning was invented in the 19th century, it was a luxury.

We still see it as a luxury. But it is a necessity if a person is in a wheelchair in a stifling apartment whose windows are nailed shut because of a justified fear of burglary or home invasion. A place to cool off may not be a luxury for a homeless person living under a viaduct or on a searing sidewalk.

The situation is especially difficult because many people who are at risk are afraid to leave their homes for cooling centers, because they fear there won't be anything left when they get back. And that assumes that they understand the risk they face, which is not always the case. Also, many of these folks simply can't afford the amount of electricity that air conditioning requires.

After the horror became obvious, the city of Chicago developed and implemented a heat emergency plan, and the number of deaths dropped to only a few in subsequent heat waves. But it should not have taken more than 700 deaths for us to realize that, just like influenza, hyperthermia is an epidemic that will sweep over us from time to time. We need to be prepared.

Let us resolve to ensure that healthcare providers are more involved in public education about heat-related illness, and that we also work to educate municipal, county, and state authorities about the danger. Providers should also have their own heat plans, so that they can be of help to those at risk. With all the talk these days about providers' desire to promote "healthy communities," we should be able to protect our neighbors from poaching to death in their own homes.

Mickey Mantle's Transplant

There will be debate for a long time over what the Baylor transplant team did wrong or right in giving a liver transplant to a celebrity who had cancer, hepatitis C, and a long history of alcoholism. The ethics journals will be full of musings on the subject, and many people will always believe that he was given special treatment because he was an American cultural icon. His physicians deny that he was "jumped" in queue or that he was a poor candidate, clinically, for a transplant; they also reject the notion that he should have been turned down because until a few months before his transplant, he had been drinking heavily for years.

All these issues are sensitive and subjective, and they will likely never be settled. The issue of queue-jumping had been raised previously in the case of organs becoming almost immediately available for Governor Casey of Pennsylvania, and it will be raised again in the future—in fact, every time a famous transplant candidate gets organs quickly. And it probably should be brought up often, just to make sure that the organ distribution system we have gone to such great pains to create remains untainted, objective, and fair.

The question of whether someone with multiple morbidities, who is known to have cancer, should receive a transplant and then be treated with large amounts of immunosuppressive drugs (which will feed any cancer that is present—and did) is, on one level, a clinical issue. The Baylor team claims that it not only met, but exceeded, clinical practice standards in terms of determining that Mantle's cancer was confined to his liver. They said the fact that the cancer had spread could only have been learned after the transplant.

But other news stories suggested that some members of the transplant team believed that evidence of other sites of cancer was there during the surgery, and that the team did the procedure anyway because "otherwise he would have died on the table," technically because his liver had been removed. The surgeons apparently could not accept that outcome.

I doubt we will ever know all that happened. But I do know that donor livers are in scarce supply in this country. I do know that 10 percent of patients waiting for donor livers die before receiving one.

I also know that healthcare must constantly balance two roles: one as protector and champion of the individual patient, and the other as steward of societal resources, which include money, buildings, skills, and donor organs. We have been entrusted by our fellow citizens with enormous amounts of power, autonomy, and especially trust; we should husband those gifts with a keen sense of responsibility and humility. We should not play fast and loose with them.

The very fact that so many questions were raised about the Baylor team's account of what happened shows that there are many in the press and the general public who are increasingly skeptical about how well we manage the trust we hold.

Let us resolve to keep in mind, at all times, that we in healthcare hold in our hands the resources and trust of all those in this country, and that we owe them honesty in return. We cannot call futile care "heroic" or "experimental." We cannot waste resources, and lives, and call it compassion. In a time when tens of millions are uninsured and our great national health programs are being cut back, we have to be very careful about what we do with what we have.

Medicaid and Medicare

There was much talk this year about the impending demise of Social Security and Medicare. (There was very little talk about Medicaid's problems.) As I write this, the air is filled with helpful suggestions as to how to resolve the crisis. These range from privatizing Medicare and turning Medicaid into a block grant to just trimming here and there to junking the whole thing.

There were also many pronouncements, in this thirtieth anniversary year, on what the programs did not do. Medicare pays only about half of the average elderly person's healthcare bills; Medicaid has never come close to protecting all the poor. The vision that these programs would be the basis for universal coverage never came to fruition, to put it mildly. All in all, Medicare is viewed as a modest success, and Medicaid as a dismal failure.

This is not true. Whatever their faults—and they are many—Medicare and Medicaid have provided healthcare protection to tens of millions of people over the past 30 years. They ended the threat of poverty for millions of senior citizens. They made good nursing home care available to people who could never have afforded it on their own. They kept end-stage renal disease from being a death sentence. They enabled massively improved quality of life for many disabled Americans. Had these programs not existed, an intolerable amount of suffering, premature death, and disability would have plagued us to this day.

Medicaid and Medicare, like Social Security before them, also represent a promise. They were the embodiment of a covenant that the people of this country made with each other during the darkest days of the Depression: that we will afford each other some degree of protection against catastrophe, even at some small cost to ourselves. What we forget, in these latter days, is that the fact that the elderly and the poor are doing better, at least in terms of access to healthcare, is not evidence that Medicare and Medicaid are unnecessary and can be cut to pieces, but is rather evidence of how well they have worked and how much they are needed.

Medicaid and Medicare had a lot to do with American healthcare getting fat and sassy in the past 30 years; it seems to me that we owe these programs, and their beneficiaries, something in return. If we make no other resolutions for the new year, let us make—and keep—this one: that we respect the social protections that Medicaid and Medicare represent, as well as the promise that they continue to hold for all of us. And although we know that they can be changed for the better, and we will strive to be part of that process, we will not allow their protections to be lost—or their promise betrayed.

Happy New Year.

A Demanding Issue

January 1996

A friend of mine who has had a long and distinguished career in health policy once told me that he had come to the saddening and bitter conclusion that the only way to achieve change in healthcare is to get the payers to force change—that is, in the end, providers will move only when their finances are at stake.

Another friend of mine, Austin Ross of the University of Washington (formerly of the Virginia Mason Medical Center in Seattle), has written that healthcare people do not tend to change unless a certain level of anxiety has been reached—otherwise they are just too comfortable to do much, even if there is pressing need.

I would add, out of my own dubious wisdom, that once providers decide that they do want to change, all too often they do so at the speed of light—heading off in the wrong direction, bumping into chairs, tripping over things, and causing all kinds of damage along the way.

These days, all three dynamics are in play: The payers are making big-time demands, providers have reached the critical mass of anxiety (actually, I think it's more like terror), and everyone from physicians to big systems is running around like a chicken that is missing part of its anatomy.

When such an environment develops, my instinctive tendency is to mutter, "Patients beware!" I have been muttering that a lot lately.

Why? Because everywhere I look, I see a shift in the basic philosophy of the patient-provider relationship. From day one in this country, that relationship has had its moral hazards, from physician paternalism and withholding of information to the overprovision of healthcare. The latter risk was the most constant.

Indeed, if one holds with the payer-as-driving-force theory, to which I reluctantly subscribe at the moment, it would figure that when the provider was paid more if he or she or it did more, the trend would be toward overcare and even marginal or useless treatment. A growing body of evidence has indicated that was the case.

There were a few voices speaking out against this excess—some of the early HMO pioneers like Sidney Garfield, MD (father of the Permanente Medical Groups), and later John Wennberg, MD, and Sidney Wolfe, MD. But for the most part, it was "the more the better."

And isn't it funny that during those halcyon days, I didn't hear anyone talking about "demand reduction" and "demand management"? Indeed, those who suggested that providing everything under the sun, regardless of whether there was any scientific basis for doing so, was potentially harmful were accused of trying to "ration care."

All of a Sudden

Now, of course, we are in the age of discounts, capitation, and the less you do, the more money you make. And all of a sudden, it's those blasted patients who keep demanding everything in sight, who insist on care that can't do them any good, who think the healthcare system can achieve miracles.

I wonder what led them to behave like that?

It certainly couldn't have been provider advertisements that promised total cures of everything from acne to heart disease. It certainly couldn't have been tens of thousands of press releases over the years issued by providers, suppliers, and pharmaceutical houses, each trying to cajole the press into reporting on another breakthrough, another miracle. It certainly couldn't have been a medical culture so afraid of "failure"—that is, patient death—that patients took to sniffing carbon monoxide in the back of a minivan rather than go on living in agony.

And, of course, it wasn't Mickey Mantle's transplant team, who, faced with a patient suffering from metastasized cancer, hepatitis C, and alcoholic cirrhosis, decided to give him a liver, anyway, and pump him full of immunosuppressives so the cancer could spread faster—and who covered their tracks by calling it "experimental therapy." Others have used less kind terms to describe it.

The sudden, widespread condemnation of "inappropriate patient demand" begins to ring a little hollow when one notices how closely it is tied to changes in financial incentives, regardless of clinical incentives—and how it disregards the fact that a great deal of patient demand was triggered by providers over the years.

Do patients demand care they don't need, care that can't help them and may even harm them? You bet they do. There are a multitude of examples:

- Guilt-stricken families who insist that an elderly relative (now in a persistent vegetative state) continue to receive "treatment"—even kidney dialysis and organ transplants—because of unresolved family issues

- Terrified parents who refuse to believe that a beloved child is beyond help

- Spouses, parents, or others who, as in the Helga Wanglie case in Minnesota, believe that "only God can take life," and interpret that belief as meaning that infinite intervention by the healthcare system, even if futile, is necessary

- Patients with failing organs or other severe conditions who seek miracles and demand long-odds therapy because they have been told there is "a chance"—as in the 1 percent odds of survival given to the parents of the conjoined Lakeberg twins (both of whom ended up

dead, one from having her heart removed and the
other from multiple causes after a year on life support)

- Patients who don't want to be inconvenienced by
minor ills or untimely events, and who, as a result, seek
antibiotics for viral infections and cesareans for perfectly normal births

- Aging or insecure patients who use extensive cosmetic
surgery and then try to find ways to get their health
insurance to pay for it (and some health insurers,
incredibly, do)

- Even the occasional felon, like the father who had
beaten his daughter to a pulp, leaving her in a persistent vegetative state, who insisted that she be kept on
life support because as long as she was technically
"alive," he wasn't guilty of murder

Stories Providers Tell Themselves

Yes, patients can and do abuse the system. But as we condemn them
roundly for doing so, stringently limiting their access so they won't
do so, and trying to convince them that they really don't want any
healthcare, let's talk about the other end of the spectrum: demand
inducement and all the stories providers have told themselves over
the years about why they offer, and provide, unnecessary care:

If I don't do it, somebody else will. I have heard this one a lot
over the years. The argument is that if a patient demands antibiotics
for a viral infection, and a physician refuses to provide them, the
patient will go somewhere else. In other words, in order to prevent
some other doctor from practicing bad medicine, I'll practice it myself.
And, by the way, I'll get the payment, and not that other, bad doctor.

It's the patient's decision. How many times, in order to avoid
accountability for the decision, has a physician or nurse or other
healthcare person provided the patient with information on every
option known to humankind, and then said, "It's up to you"? This

occurs even when some of the options are ridiculous. Physicians would claim it was their solemn duty to offer the patient everything, even if it was the longest of shots. But as physician Leslie Blackhall has written, if something won't do any good, the provider is under no imperative to offer it. Why, she asks, do we continue to use CPR on patients who can't benefit from it? The operative philosophy seems to be a healthcare corollary of the Edmund Hillary "Everest Principle": Use it because it's there.

They'll sue me. Of course, a fear of malpractice litigation is the handiest of excuses for inducing patient demand. Although over-aggressive, money-hungry attorneys have made a shambles of what should be a patient protection activity, it is also true that most true malpractice cases are never litigated, and that there is something called the "standard of care"—that is, if the physician or hospital adhered to the prevailing standard of treatment in that community, he, she, or it is not guilty of malpractice. It is going to be interesting to see how long it takes malpractice attorneys to start suing HMOs and PPOs, as opposed to physicians, for not doing this or that. (Actually, they've already started.)

It might work. Despite all the precautions—ethics committees, institutional review boards, standards and protocols, second opinions—there are still those who see every patient as a potential research subject who might be suitable for a little experimentation. Indeed, the argument is often raised that if we don't "push the envelope" (how I hate that phrase!), we'll never learn anything. As a result, all kinds of really dubious care—particularly involving organ transplantation, potentially harmful pharmaceuticals, and "heroic" treatment of dread disease—are carried on under the umbrella of research. Keep in mind that this is the same term used by the Nazi doctors in the camps to describe their work.

The Nature of Demand

So maybe it isn't just patients who make inappropriate demands; maybe it's decades of the healthcare system inducing demand in them. And maybe we should think twice about slamming on the brakes and charging off in precisely the opposite direction, seeing how little we can get away with providing, just because that's where the financial incentives have moved.

Maybe, in fact, we should think about some of the underlying principles that should govern any attempts to raise, lower, or change the nature of demand for healthcare:

Abandonment. Healthcare philosopher Daniel Callahan, whom I have quoted before in this regard, explained years ago that when patients fear abandonment by the healthcare system—usually because they are dying, or chronically ill, or have a disease that is not "interesting" to physicians—they will try to stay in the acute-care sector and demand more and more treatment, simply because they don't want to be left lying by the side of the road. If we could develop more respect for nonacute, nonglamorous patients and their conditions, a great deal of inappropriate demand would dissipate.

Fear of too-tight limits. As I predicted, we are now seeing a backlash against managed care plans that constrain access too tightly. The battle that emerged in 1995 over "drive-through births"— discharging mothers and their newborns in eight or 12 hours, without their consent—has led to a flood of legislation designed to protect the patients involved. It is only the first of what will be many fights, as managed care moves beyond capturing helpless, politically powerless welfare families to placing severe limits on the access of privately insured middle-class patients, who can and will fight back. And every time a fight like this breaks out, nervous patients can be expected to question every turn-down of a request more strongly as they wonder if the decision was clinical or economic.

Lack of objective standards. Although it is in its infancy, the movement toward objective clinical standards that are scientifically derived (as opposed to being based on economic or malpractice concerns) will do much to alleviate what is one of our two biggest problems: the fact that much of the time, we do not know what works and what does not. As a result, a great deal of healthcare constitutes a shot in the dark. This produces unnecessary care, harm to patients, and needless expense. However, it is not much of an improvement to deny care in the same haphazard, maybe-it-won't-hurt-and-might-help manner. I personally tend to think that, in a marginal situation, not doing something is preferable to doing something. But that's not always best. We don't know what is best. We need to redouble our efforts to find out.

Oversupply. This is the other big problem: We have too many hospitals, too many specialist physicians, maybe too many nurses (I'm not convinced of that), and too many practitioners of virtually every health profession, up to and including administrators. As a result, there is a constant threat of lower incomes, underemployment, unemployment, bankruptcy, and closure. Providers will do whatever is necessary to keep functioning and to achieve that target income, whether it is setting up boutique practices near HMO clinics to catch dissatisfied patients who didn't get what they wanted (even if they didn't need it), or establishing transplant programs that could not possibly do enough procedures to be good at it, or developing wacky new therapies aimed at intractable conditions such as AIDS or malignant melanoma.

John Wennberg said it several years ago: If we do not turn down, in his words, "the supply thermostat" to some reasonable level, even capitation and discounts and extremely tight managed care will not prevent providers from doing what is not needed—and talking patients into going along with it.

The issues of demand reduction, demand management, and demand inducement are all the same issue, and they all have the same ultimate resolution: We need to learn what works in healthcare; we need to learn what patients want when presented with information about all the useful and appropriate options; and we need to gain the discipline to live with the results of that knowledge. Blaming patients for decades of excess in the healthcare system will not solve our problems.

Articles Not Included

S ix articles by the author that were published in *Healthcare Forum* and *Healthcare Forum Journal* were not included in this volume.

"Room at the Top" (January 1986): This article did not address ethics, but rather women in health administration, and is badly outdated.

"What Do Consumers Really Want?" (May 1986): Similarly, this was not an ethics piece, but rather an examination of healthcare consumerism.

"Ethics as a Community Project" (March 1988): This piece discussed a series of community ethics projects that have long since ended.

"Managing Ethics in Managed Care" (March 1989): This topic was addressed in a more detailed and thorough piece in 1993, which is included in this volume.

"Color, Consciousness, and Change" (May 1989): This piece, which focused on race and related issues, contained a large amount of data that are now badly out of date.

"America's Growing Diversity" (January 1992): This article did not concern ethics, but was rather written for a special issue on demographic diversity.

Index

About The Author

Emily Friedman is a Chicago-based health policy and ethics analyst and lecturer. She is a contributing editor of *Healthcare Forum Journal*, *Hospitals and Health Networks*, and the "Policy Watch" section of the *American Journal of Medicine*. She is also an adjunct assistant professor at the Boston University School of Public Health, where she teaches a graduate course in rationing and resource allocation in health care. From September 1987 to June 1988, she was a Rockefeller Fellow in Ethics at Dartmouth College, Hanover, New Hampshire.

She is originally from Los Angeles and graduated with honors from the University of California at Berkeley in 1968.